Perspectives on Care at Home for Older People

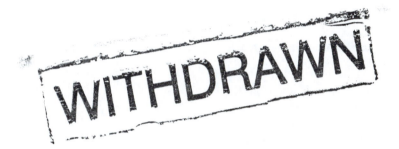

Routledge Studies in Health and Social Welfare

Perspectives on Care at Home for Older People

**Edited by Christine Ceci,
Kristín Björnsdóttir and
Mary Ellen Purkis**

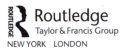
Routledge
Taylor & Francis Group
NEW YORK   LONDON

First published 2012
by Routledge
711 Third Avenue, New York, NY 10017

Simultaneously published in the UK
by Routledge
2 Park Square, Milton Park, Abingdon, Oxon OX14 4RN

*Routledge is an imprint of the Taylor & Francis Group,
an informa business*

© 2012 Taylor & Francis

The right of Christine Ceci, Kristín Björnsdóttir and Mary Ellen Purkis to
be identified as the authors of the editorial material, and of the authors for
their individual chapters, has been asserted in accordance with sections 77
and 78 of the Copyright, Designs and Patents Act 1988.

Typeset in Sabon by IBT Global.

First issued in paperback 2013

Library of Congress Cataloging-in-Publication Data

Perspectives on care at home for older people / edited by Christine Ceci,
    Kristin Björnsdóttir, and Mary Ellen Purkis.
      p. ; cm. — (Routledge studies in health and social welfare ; 6)
    Includes bibliographical references and index.
      1. Older people—Home care. I. Ceci, Christine. II. Kristín
Björnsdóttir. III. Purkis, Mary Ellen. IV. Series: Routledge studies
in health and social welfare ; 6.
    [DNLM: 1. Home Care Services. 2. Aged. 3. Health Services for
the Aged. 4. Long-Term Care—methods. WY 115.1]
    RA645.35.P47 2011
    362.14—dc23
    2011008959

ISBN: 978-0-415-84989-0 (pbk)
ISBN: 978-0-415-89590-3 (hbk)
ISBN: 978-0-203-80567-1 (ebk)

Nothing should be more expected than old age: nothing is more unforeseen.

—Simone de Beauvoir, *The Coming of Age*

Contents

PART III
Practices

Foreword

Illness is a Plural—Home Care, Governmentality and Reframing the Work of Patienthood

Carl May

Editors' note: Professor May's welcome contribution to this book is, uncharacteristically for a foreword, not a comment on the book itself or its contents. Rather it takes the role of context setting. Almost simultaneous with our initial meetings to determine the shape of this project, the editors of this book, as well as several of the contributors, participated in a conference[1] where Dr. May delivered a plenary address, *Agency, Prudence, Expertise and Resourcefulness: Sickness Work in the 21st Century.* In this talk he sketched out certain of the forces— including epidemiological and demographic transitions—influencing current trends in the organization and delivery of health care in advanced economies and described the effects of these changes in terms of a shift in the burden of the work of illness care from providers to patients. There is, he suggested, a "wholesale re-arrangement of the work of being sick" and we ignore these structural shifts at our "peril." Well, we thought, a shifting burden of work also describes much of what we see for the older people with whom we are specifically concerned—there is also 'work' involved in being old, being frail, in needing care—and we need to be carefully attending to the way in which this is occurring. So in a sense, Dr. May sets out, in this foreword but more extensively in his other work, the problematic with which each contributor to this book grapples—the conditions of possibility for good care. (CC, KB, MEP)

Underpinning many current debates in health care is the sense that health care is at a crossroads, and that this crossroads defines more than the problems of demography and costs that policy makers—on both sides of the Atlantic—sometimes seek to make the focus of our attention. Indeed, the current healthcare crisis can be characterized as the price that the advanced economies must pay for successfully overwhelming the mass of infectious and acute disease that winnowed their populations until the mid-twentieth century (Holman 2006). Nevertheless, in those same advanced economies these successes are infrequently celebrated by policy-makers, who see in place of those winnowed generations an ever-growing cohort of older people with multiple chronic co-morbidities, who require care over lifetime illness careers, in place of cure for episodes of acute disease. The policy problem is therefore composed of a set of anxieties about the management of increasingly scarce healthcare resources, in the face of ever-growing demands. There is a sub-text to this, too. It is that sick older people are a problem because they subtract tax-dollars from the interests of younger healthy people.

In the face of these shifts, health-care researchers are often pressed to see their task as contributing to the management of scarcity (perhaps by finding rational and ethical bases for rationing and for the withdrawal of care), and to respond to this continually growing demand on social resources by finding technological fixes for it (perhaps by redirecting it into new professional or organizational systems of practice). Governmentality in contemporary healthcare is expressed, therefore, in patterns of technogovernance at the micro-scale (May et al. 2006), and in the reformulation of professional-patient relations through incremental bureaucratization and the corporate impulses of healthcare providers at the macro-scale (May 2007). In this short essay, I want to make three claims about the effects of these processes on the practices of healthcare and speak to the necessity of theory through which these effects can be defined and interpreted.

Our starting point must be the traditional way of thinking about patient-hood, in which the patient is assigned a role in relation *to* clinical practices and their contexts. Whether we see this *relation to* in terms of a very passive role or, at the other end of the spectrum, as a very active consumer of healthcare, this is a view that relies on the application of old asymmetries of power and knowledge. This is equally true of both the Parsonian assumptions underpinning 'sick role' theory (Parsons 1951, 1975) and of more recent postmodern accounts (Fox 1993; Morris 1998). Here, psyche and soma are objects to be measured and manipulated through interactions with medical knowledge and practice. But as treatments become ever more complex, and the burden of labor and time that they present to patients becomes more demanding, we need to think about the divisions between professionals and patients, between the healthy and the sick, and the sick and their significant others. This is because of the increasing burden of technical expertise, self-monitoring, self-care and routine symptom management, record-keeping and the accumulation of information, and organizational and coordinating labor that is being shifted from the clinic into the home (May 2009). Here the population of individualized patients provides an insufficient workforce to perform the business of healthcare; work has to be further distributed to family and friends as new machines are incorporated into the home, web-interfaces opened up, and telecare systems operationalized. We can find a generative principle of the emergent forms of home care at work here:

The patient is not enough.

(The burden of illness now demands more than a co-operative patient, instead it requires a compliant network.)

If the patient is not enough for healthcare systems, then the work of self-care and healthcare is an ever-expanding universe of labor. Parsons (1965) argued that we should see sickness as a "job of work" and that is precisely what it has come to be. While older people with multiple chronic co-morbidities are claimed to be a drain on resources and a brake on national economic competitiveness, they too are drained, as substantial burdens of work are shifted to them.

Of course, the work of sickness has permeable boundaries, multiple contingencies of practice, and it radically alters biographies and identities (Bury 1982; Charmaz 2006). One way of seeing this problem has been, from the earliest days of social science analysis, by applying the notion of *illness career.* Chronic illnesses are managed and modified over lifetime trajectories. They ebb and flow, suffer instabilities and exacerbations, but are equally frequently experienced as the constant and barely changing background radiation of a limiting universe. If we think again about the experience as illness, we can see these careers not as evidence of the inevitable failure of the body, but as a series of episodes of sickness engaged with implementation projects, in which different assemblages of actors and actants—drawn out of multiple territories and trajectories—are committed to the business of care. These projects multiply the possibilities of treatment and add steadily to its burden because they fragment experiences of care and threaten the individualization of patient care upon which many of the claims of professional ideologies rest. This leads us to a second generative principle:

Illness is a plural.

(In a world defined by multiple chronic co-morbidities, sickness is experienced as an assemblage of management projects rather than a phenomenological unity.)

Now, the spatial and temporal fragmentation of care means that relations between sick people and the sources of their care are often unstable and emergent, not simply because of the regularities of titration, but because of changing constructs of evidence and the timetabling of careers and credentials. We therefore need *minimally disruptive* healthcare and to consider the burden of illness in relation to the burdens and incivilities imposed on people by the proliferation and expansion of treatments, and fragmented and uncoordinated patterns in the delivery of care (May et al. 2009b). The practices of self-care, home care, and formally defined professional care are organized, increasingly, around the multiplication of coordinating activity. This takes us to a third generative principle.

The co-ordination of co-ordination is not a paradox.

(The multiplication of co-ordination gives recognition to the complexity of contemporary healthcare.)

In these contexts the *home* as the center of home care is no longer a bounded domestic territory, but is now a suburb of the healthcare system itself. It has organizational significance as a place to which clinically defined work can be relocated, and it is this—rather than any ideological or ethical impulse—that gives truth to the claim that patients are partners in their care. *Of course* patients are 'involved' in their care. They and their significant others are enrolled as unpaid workers in these extended and extending systems of practice. They contribute not only practice (doing or not doing what they are asked by health professionals), but by building a body of technical expertise that is circulated through epistemological communities that exist in parallel to, and sometimes competition with, the repositories of clinical knowledge and practice to which they are supposed to defer.

Because of the empirical shifts that I have sketched out above, we can now dispose of two analytic conventions. First, that accounting for experiences of illness and its meanings—and the biographical disruptions that stem from it—means that our analytic narratives must be primarily focused on the phenomenology of sickness. Second, that accounts of experiences of illness are an adequate response to the assumption of scarcity and the problem of rationing. The phenomenology of illness and the problem of scarcity are, it seems, united by the work that sick people and their others do to stay on top of their symptoms, to stay engaged with their treatments, and to co-ordinate and manage the combined burdens of illness and care. Theories of socio-technical change have a good deal to offer us as we attempt to understand the shift to home care because they refuse to divide the social and technical, and because they also refuse to play out the technical as either determined or determining. Home care is not the necessary outcome of cost control but is rather the product of multiple contingencies. It is one of a number of possible results of interactions between the 'social' and the 'technical', in part because this shift is an epiphenomenon of deeper and more fundamental changes in the way that healthcare systems themselves deal with the problems of coordinating coordination, of the plurality of illness and the inadequacy of patient-hood.

Where do the three generative principles that I have outlined above take us? One place that they might take us is into the domain of the *socio-technical* as it is outlined in Science and Technology Studies (Webster 2007). This is where I and my colleagues have been building theory that seeks to explain the how 'innovations' (defined broadly) are implemented, embedded and integrated in practice by healthcare providers—and the ways that the management of health technologies (again defined broadly) in practice is increasingly distributed (May and Finch 2009; May et al. 2009a). The point of emphasis here is that the more that we have examined the practices of healthcare technologies and organizations, the more we have observed the collapsing boundaries between patient, carer, worker and professional. Their work is being redistributed within compliant networks. This redistribution parallels the collection and systematization of knowledge about the health of the self and assumes a diffuse (and increasingly, unpaid) labor force. In relation to which, assumptions about the ownership of knowledge and practice can be designed *out* of artifacts and systems, as well as designed *into* them.

NOTES

1. *Government of the self in the clinic and the community,* 3rd International In Sickness & In Health Conference, April 15–17, 2009, Victoria, British Columbia, Canada.

REFERENCES

Bury, Michael. 1982. Chronic illness as biographical disruption. *Sociology of Health and Illness* 4: 167–182.

Charmaz, Kathy. 2006. *Good days, bad days: The self in chronic illness.* New Brunswick, NJ: Rutgers University Press.

Fox, Nick J. 1993. *Postmodernism, sociology and health.* Buckingham: Open University Press.

Holman, Halsted R. 2006. Chronic illness and the healthcare crisis. *Chronic Illness* 1(4): 265–274.

May, Carl. 2007. The clinical encounter and the problem of context. *Sociology* 41(1): 29–45.

——— 2009. Mundane medicine, therapeutic relationships, and the clinical encounter. In *Handbook of the sociology of health, illness, and healing: A blueprint for the 21st century,* edited by Bernice Pescosolido, Jack A. Martin, Jane McLeod and Anne Rogers, 309–322. New York: Springer.

May, Carl, and Tracy Finch. 2009. Implementation, embedding, and integration: an outline of Normalization Process Theory. *Sociology* 43(3): 535–554.

May, Carl, Frances Mair, Tracy Finch, Anne MacFarlane, Christopher Dowrick, Shaun Treweek, Tim Rapley, Luciana Ballini, Bie Nio Ong, Anne Rogers, Elizabeth Murray, Glyn Elwyn, Frances Legare, Jane Gunn and Victor Montori. 2009a. Development of a theory of implementation and integration: Normalization Process Theory. *Implementation Science* 4(29): 1–9.

May, Carl, Victor Montori, and Frances Mair. 2009b. We need minimally disruptive medicine. *BMJ* 339: b2803.

May, Carl, Tim Rapley, Tiago Moreira, Tracy Finch and B. Heaven. 2006. Technogovernance: evidence, subjectivity, and the clinical encounter in primary care medicine. *Social Science & Medicine* 62(4): 1022–1030.

Morris, D. B. 1998. *Illness and culture in the postmodern age.* London: University of California Press.

Parsons, Talcott. 1951. *The social system.* London: Routledge & Kegan Paul.

——— 1965. *Social structure and personality.* New York: Free Press.

——— 1975. The sick role and the role of the physician reconsidered. *Action Theory and the Human Condition.* New York: Free Press.

Webster, Andrew. 2007. *Health, technology and society: A sociological critique.* Basingstoke: Palgrave Macmillan.

Introduction

Home, Care, Practice—Changing Perspectives on Care at Home for Older People

Christine Ceci, Kristín Björnsdóttir and Mary Ellen Purkis

Conceiving of a thing is a fundamental kind of political activity.
—Alan Finlayson, 2006

Library shelves all over the Western world are heavily weighted with books that take up questions of the 'problems' of age and what should be done about it. Standing in front of these shelves can be not only intimidating but also a little bit disheartening. Row upon row of handbooks on age and ageing written for nurses, social workers, gerontologists, psychologists, sociologists and families going back decades. Books by and for researchers, academics, bureaucrats, practitioners and the general public. National surveys and outcomes research line up beside personal accounts, analyses of political and economic implications rest against organizational strategies for providing efficient services, assessments of the effects of health system restructuring crowd out guides intended to assist families to cope with their care 'burden'. This 'problem'—becoming old and what to do about that—has clearly, and for some time, preoccupied many. Surely by now everything critical, instructional or reflective has already been said. And yet it has not because, evidently, we still struggle with the question of how we want this to proceed, this caring for frail older adults in our societies.

This question of how to respond to the perceived challenges of ageing populations is very much on the policy and research agenda of many nations, and significant discussions are occurring concerning the place of formal home care, its possibilities and limitations, in meeting these challenges. Yet home care, as a formal practice, remains significantly under-theorized, with the meanings and assumptions shaping its key concepts—home, care and practice—rarely made explicit. Home care as such is assumed to require neither explanation nor analysis. Yet as a field of care, home care is made up of much that is materially and meaningfully heterogeneous. Discourses highlighting vulnerability, frailty or a decline associated with ageing run up against a rhetoric of self-reliance, responsibility and independence; those highlighting supply, demand and scarcity of resources push back against claims of justice or entitlement—and vice versa. And the 'field' itself is contested, complex and dispersed, spread as it is across multiple, often hidden locations of activity (Baranek, Deber, and Williams 2004). A shift in the preferred site of care from hospital to people's homes has implications for experiences of home and care and for the organization of the work itself. In many locations, there are disputes about the prioritization of different types of clients with different types of needs, concerns about resources spread too thinly, and apprehension about the effects of discourses of responsibilization and individualization and the growing influence of neo-liberal discourses in delimiting the role of the state. Yet in this mix and mess of discourses and practices, a complexity reflective of most areas of modern life, there remains, somewhere at home care's core, the matter of concern of this practice—the enormously important questions people have about how they are going to be able to live their lives.

This collection is informed by this concern and framed by two central questions that examine the line currently taken around home-based supportive care and services for 'frail' older people. How do the actualities of people's daily lives articulate with ideological, practical and programmatic discourses and material conditions? And what are the conditions of possibility for 'care' where the frailties of older people matter? And because in this collection we are most concerned with the organization of formal home care, within these central questions lurk many others: What is the state's role in supporting those who are older and frail? What justifies or explains state involvement in or detachment from the 'private' life of citizens? These latter questions offer opportunities for thinking through not only what we mean by and require from the state but also, and reciprocally, how state-sponsored processes and practices function to constitute us as particular kinds of citizens. In some locations, Canada and the UK for example, it seems that it has become increasingly difficult to simply assert that people need to be cared for, a claim somewhat less contentious in the context of the Nordic welfare state—though here too, this ethic of care is changing. But increasingly, the argument must actually be made that those who are older and frail need help or assistance with various activities so they can lead a satisfying life. It seems that in these situations, where there are fewer clear links with the taken-for-granted constituents of appropriate health services, more convincing strategies of justification must be developed to support the provision of what comes to be called 'social' care, or care that helps people to hold on to the life they are living (see Ceci and Purkis 2011). This is a location of care that we think requires a more sustained theorizing: how are the boundaries between those who do and do not need help constituted and maintained?

The contributors to this collection write from a range of disciplinary backgrounds and geopolitical contexts demonstrating at the very least that home care is mediated by the settings in which it is enacted, with the particulars of practices shaped by local policies, priorities and resources.

International comparisons that theorize the social organization of home care bring to the fore deeply held views of what such help looks like and how it may be accomplished. As Kari Waerness (2005) argues, examining work that is contextual and descriptive contributes to understanding what is specific to providing good care. Attention to the specificity of diverse contexts also enables analysis of the ways that local social, economic and political systems and structures influence our views of the possible, and in so doing, enlarges these views. So though contributors to this volume do not develop prescriptions for practice, they articulate knowledge of the conditions of possibility for providing home care, that is, how current arrangements produce divisions among people, health and social care and the ways these are linked to a whole range of external influences and relations.

In Conversation[1] (1)

Davina Allen: So having done some critique of this business of home-based care, what can be done? I'm feeling like I want to be able to do something differently, and recognizing how problematic that is; like, is it possible? Just feeling like I can't stay here [with critique only] for too much longer, because it's just too uncomfortable. . . . So on what basis can I engage in that sort of writing or action with local health authorities or whomever to make these sorts of practices be more amenable and more sensitive and more permission granting. . . .

Mary Ellen Purkis: When I think about the paper I've written for this [meeting] and my interest in home care, and my interest in the kinds of questions Christine has raised for me about how do we want this to proceed, this kind of caring for frail older adults in our society, and I think about my parents as a sort of instance of that case . . . and the very brute force kind of way that we have to do this work seems so wrong against who these people are and what it might be that they're looking for. . . . In the literatures we are all most familiar with, is it the case that critiques have been undertaken, and then things have just been sort of left? So that we've got all of this—we've got this analysis of all the issues that face us, but there's not as much—okay, so what can we do about this now, what are the matters of concern. . . .

Sirpa Wrede: I think it would be very difficult for us as a group [to devise a programmatic intervention] . . . even though we would be *willing* to make a program for good care, I think we are coming from different contexts, we would be talking about different things when we would come down to the detail. . . . But I think what I've been getting from the discussion so far is that what we share is a sense of the devaluation of care and the need to tackle that kind of analysis. We are trying to talk about normative issues without becoming programmatic ... and yet I think that a risk of the use of the concept of care is that you tend to make the people objects of care and voiceless. ... I think that perhaps we could try to think about frailty as a basis of social division, a way of othering and try to address how that takes place when we talk about care: how do we end up othering the older people who are in need of these services?

Joanna Latimer: One of the things that is so interesting about what you are saying is the idea that "we've got to go to the old," because we are always thinking of it in this dyadic relation. I mean, they're as much participants as anybody else. They may lie low and efface themselves but they're still participating in particular kinds of practices and processes. So it's not to give them voice; it's the older person as a participant in this process ... however, this idea of frailty, some think of frailty as something that inheres in persons, frailty and helplessness; but that's a relational effect. ... the minute you flip the world by saying that what frailty is is not just something that inheres in somebody because they can't see, they can't hear, they can't walk. ... It's this relation between this body and the world in which they live, once you flip that over, you rescue the old immediately—they get rescued and brought back into play.

Sirpa Wrede: I think we need to think more about the concept of frailty somehow, I'm thinking of frailty as a social division that can be analyzed like other divisions such as gender. Not talking against how you are deconstructing frailty but holding on to the fact that it really is relevant in the way we talk about people. And I think a similar issue for me would be work, the position of home care work as devalued work is influenced by cultural understandings of old age ... that is then how I go to the notion of power ...

Christine Ceci: These are ideas that we have each committed to drawing through our papers, about practices and the effects of practices and how practices constitute particular realities, and how power is relevant in all of that. These are questions that people take up differently but they have a place in everyone's approach around the general idea of how do we—so much of the language of this has become more and more problematic-but how do we provide 'care' for people who are older and frail and needing *something*. ... But that's why we are thinking in terms of frailty ... there're reasons why these people are there, are involved. Is it a matter of the distinction being that these are practices that aren't oriented to fixing people, that there's an ongoing-ness to the practices that are initiated because of frailty of some sort?

Mary Ellen Purkis: What I kind of like about it actually, the concept of frailty, is that it's—it isn't something that can be fixed, it's only something that can be supported. You can support people who are frail to be a little less frail; you can't fix it . . . which is maybe what a lot of home care practice is trying but failing to do.

Hanne Marlene Dahl: There is a sense that the configurations of the elderly and the home helper, they don't seem to fit, and the reason that they don't fit is that the [policy] discourse, when it articulates the elderly person, it very much continues this 'will to the pleasant', which is sort of a pun on Foucault's will to power . . . all the positive, good things in the elderly get articulated whereas all the fragility and all the sadness disappears. So there is this will to the pleasant where strength and empowerment and self-determination are strongly articulated and all the other things are silenced.

HOME

And this is the allure of home care: the home as a pleasant, comfortable, comforting, healing space, as though the space itself would do a good bit of the work that is required by frail elders. But home is a contested and diverse space (Yanzi and Rosenberg 2008). For some it offers the familiarity and support of well-known nooks and corners, a place surrounded by neighbors who keep a respectful 'eye' on one another; for others home represents a dangerous and isolating prison where only luck reveals an individual in desperate need of care and support. Home can be as inhospitable a space as the most unreconstituted asylums of the distant past. In and of itself, it cannot heal. But networked with people and services and an ethos of concern for others, a supportive environment can emerge (Coles 1999).

Each of the contributors to this volume has approached their research in full recognition of these contestations regarding home and each takes up the perspective of those for whom care in the home is of concern. For instance, Davina Allen (this volume) examines the ways in which hospital staff mediate opportunities for hospitalized patients to return to their homes, with or without formal supports, to rehabilitate following hospitalization or, indeed, to simply pick up their lives where they left off prior to hospitalization. Allen's paper demonstrates an interesting and potentially problematic gap in understanding the extent to which frail older adults and those living with significant chronic illness function more effectively within their own home environment than may be evident in the institutional context. By contrast, Hanne Marlene Dahl (this volume) approaches the topic from the perspective of policy makers who have responsibilities for establishing standards for service provision and ensuring accountability for the expenditure of public funds. Dahl's chapter demonstrates the effects and impacts imposed through a discourse of quality rather than care for those charged with providing assistance to frail elders living in the community, as well as for the experience of that care provision.

These chapters offer eloquent insights into the tensions that become apparent when the oppositions of home as prison and home as space of healing are explicitly drawn. The ideas expressed here stimulate questions, and give consideration to just how much surveillance any one person is willing to subject themselves to in order to ensure that early signs of slow decline will be noticed and acted upon in an appropriate way. The chapters also allow us to give consideration to both how and where home-based care may transform a frail elder's daily experience of life from *quality* into *endurance*.

What can we learn from these descriptions and analyses? One outcome is most notable and that is that the idea of 'home' can no longer be taken at face value. For, as Joanna Latimer (this volume) sets out, we should not confuse the idea of 'home' for the house where we live. Indeed, Latimer focuses on precisely those situations whereby people make themselves at home—anywhere! And, in thinking of home *this* way, we can at least partially detach from the notion of a built space when we think of care at home: Latimer's contribution encourages us to think *as well* about the possibilities of enabling people to *be* at home—in spaces *beyond* their own empirical 'homes'.

In drawing our attention to such insights and offering us new ways to think about the possibilities and challenges confronting us all as we seek to live meaningfully as we age, the contributors to this volume advance the dialogue about home care and care for the elderly. The efforts taken during our time together to acknowledge with respect the critical literature on home care that we advance from, the way that literature has tended to focus on the disproportionate and negative impact that home care programs have on women (see Armstrong, Armstrong and Scott-Dixon 2008; Benoit and Hallgrimsdottir 2011, Williams and Crooks 2008). In the conversation that follows, readers will hear the points of departure that the contributions in this volume take from that base.

In Conversation (2)

> *Mary Ellen Purkis:* So I thought, "what is it about a home that would make it be a place for somebody where they would want to be cared for? What are the considerations?" Most of what

I read that comes out of healthcare and nursing on community is the happy community, the helpful community, the goodness of community . . . and it doesn't necessarily appeal to me. A lot of the people that I worry about who are frail, it doesn't seem to me like it would be a very solid thing to imagine that the community was going to look after you, and I think that that's probably *not* most people's experience these days. . . .

Joanna Latimer: I'm very interested in people, how some people can make themselves at home anywhere. I'm very interested in getting rid of the idea of home being your house. I think that's something we're positioned into very much at the moment: you own your own home; your own home is a space of identity, work and consumption, and all the rest of it; it's another cultural performance. So I'm very interested this idea that home isn't a site of ontological security, home is something people make together.

Sirpa Wrede: They're starting to look back at the situation in Finland in the late 1990s, after a recession with very heavy cuts being implemented in home care. It became a powerful experience—finding out we were looking at a loss of a knowledge base in the Nordic context, in terms of there having existed an investment in what we called *socially defined care* . . . meaning that the starting point for home care was helping the person to hold onto their lifestyle of choice for as long as possible in a home context, if that was their wish. Because for a long time, residential care was not considered to be something to be avoided with every means, but there was also the option for home care—before what you could identify as neo-liberal reforms.

Kristin Björnsdottir: Studying the history of nursing in Iceland, I found so many instances where home care had been flourishing, so I wondered why from the middle of the 20th century, there was almost no mention of home care. As I was doing this, I was reading literature from other countries where there was this call for home care—that wasn't really happening in Iceland because the Icelandic nation is still quite young and we had a lot of nursing homes, so basically that was the way to do it in Iceland—when the time has come, we go to a nursing home. But I was reading this literature and becoming more and more critical about all this work being dumped on women: what is it going to mean for them and for the future. And now there is this reframing of the situation where all of a sudden, things that used to be the responsibility of the state—you know, coming from a Nordic culture where the notion of the welfare state is so strong. And this discourse is creeping in everywhere: "No, it's not our responsibility as a society, it's the family's responsibility." That made me really worried about the nurses. The nurses in Iceland were, "Yes, this is so good. It's so good for people to be living in their own homes. Of course, it *should* be the family taking care of these people, of *course*."

Joanna Latimer: There's this alignment between the reorganization of health services and the idea that institutions are bad . . . this idea that you need to be home to be happy. So just to pick up your point that the nurses said "of course!"—so did everybody in part because there has been an erosion of this idea of institutions which is married to the idea of self-determination, autonomy and choice being all that we need.

Isabel Dyck: When you're looking at care being given in the home, it's a very hidden workplace, and that causes all sorts of dilemmas for both the caregivers and the care recipients. People talk about what they know is allowed and what isn't. There's a case where the homemaker said, "I'm not allowed to clean the windows. But this person sits by the window, and her whole life is looking out the window to see what's going on; that's her quality of life under very restrictive circumstances." So she said, "I clean the window because I see that as a health need, not a social need." But in doing so, care providers put in unpaid hours or their job may be at risk. So I think when you are talking about discretion, or accommodation . . . how do you protect the care provider as well as the care recipient. . .?

Joanna Latimer: It's very difficult to walk away. Once you've noticed—once you've noticed the window and all—I am not saying it's true in all cases; I'm just saying *when* it occurs, that kind of attention, the recognition of something, it's very hard—how do you walk away from it once you've noticed?

Isabel Dyck: In terms of home, I think that it is very clear that in different cultural contexts . . . in different countries or between people of different social classes, home can be seen as a very middle class project in terms of the way you [Joanna] were talking about identity work—and historically, it's been a middle-class privilege to have a home. So I think in terms of the privacy of the home, the intimacy of home, what home means . . . I think you could find very different meanings. When we are talking about home, we are probably talking about the construction of home and trying to be aware of home as something that is made.

Joanna Latimer: [Marilyn] Strathern, when she is writing about anthropology at home, she says, "How would we know when we are at home?" What does that mean, to think about home being a space of care?

Isabel Dyck: I guess you could look at what we're doing as elaborating on the way that homes are brought into being as a site of care, because homes, the whole concept of homes is fluid. We can think of it as a discursive field that has expectations of often, family relations, which is often the nuclear family. It's interesting to look at the social/political construction of the home, which seems to have specific functions attached to it; it's written into policy about where care should take place, which obviously will interweave with those dimensions of home that the person living in a particular dwelling brings to that. So I think what has been pointed out already is that the meaning of home is not the same for everybody. So very different sites, but it will have meanings; it's also a very practical, concrete place that has certain features to it. . . . There's a spatiality to this understanding, or as Foucault talked about, the spatialization of the medical gaze, and the possibility that we're looking at home as another site that is part of this medicalization of space. . . . I think one of the things too, about homes is the boundaries are fluid, so when home care is thought about, it's about this abstract idea of home, which of course is located in a neighborhood, in a particular city, in a region, which will have possibly quite different resources around it. So you're not necessarily just looking at that one home, but everything that is necessary to it. And for the providers, we asked them why, and all of them say, "It is so rewarding this work, hard though it is, the reward of allowing someone to stay in their own home."

Davina Allen: There's something in what you said, though, that maintaining someone in their own home, that's the end, that's what's intrinsically rewarding and I think that speaks volumes in terms of the value to be cared for in your own home has assumed in terms of this bigger issue about how do you look after people who are frail . . .

Joanna Latimer: The idea that home is the place where you can make decisions, you make choices, you can be yourself, it's something you have, it's your own. So the way we think of home is very much figured within that set of relations that produces the individual, the autonomous individual . . . so much of our policy is playing this card. So what we were thinking about is how can we get ourselves out of that. . . . One of the things I was thinking through in this paper, which I think a number of you are also raising, is for home to be a space of care, it has to be about much more than mere existence on the one side, and it actually has to be about much more than just choices and individual respect on the other—you have to have those things, but it has to be about more than that.

CARE

Home care, as the term indicates, refers to activity or work that is performed to assist someone living in his or her home. It has its roots in unpaid and often invisible work of women which in many countries, particularly in the Nordic countries, was re-defined to some extent as the responsibility of the welfare state in the latter part of the twentieth century (Holter 1984). This work has been the focus of attention in the feminist literature since the 1970s. It is often described as a labor of love, an activity that unites the work involved in caring for someone and the emotions related to caring about someone (Finch and Groves 1983). By making the complexity, effort and emotional strain involved in caring visible, feminists tried to raise public awareness around its importance to society (Fisher and Tronto 1990).

Care and caring became the focus of feminist theorizing with the publication of influential works in the 1980s, such as Carol Gilligan's *In a different voice,* where the ethical aspects of care were emphasized (Gilligan 1982). Later these theories were criticized for ignoring the antagonisms or conflicts that often arise in relationships (Cloyes 2002), for being insensitive to the imbalance of power in the way in which the caring relationship is conceptualized (Watson et al. 2004), and for a largely sanitized and idealized approach to human connection (Cooper 2007). Rather than working from the accepted feminist ethical approach, Davina Cooper developed a non-normative analysis of care. Her theorization was based on fieldwork conducted in Toronto women's bathhouses, which extends the traditional understanding of caring in important ways. In the bathhouse, caring was not mostly driven by relationships of intimacy, affection or responsibility, the key ideas in most theories on caring. Caring was provided because things and people mattered to the participants. Another key idea was attentiveness. As Cooper explains: "Attentiveness demands . . . a highly attuned sensitivity to one's environment, especially to subtle and changing complex cues, and to 'backroom' and more obscured goings on" (Cooper 2007, 255–256). This is not confined to the way in which individuals act but can be the way in which organizations operate, that is, part of organizational practices.

Davina Cooper's insights are important because caregiving in the home has, in many countries, been transformed from being provided as unpaid labor by family or friends to being a formal service provided by someone who is at least in the first place a stranger to the person being cared for. In the Nordic countries in particular, in developments described as women friendly, the public sector took over many of women's traditional responsibilities in the family, allowing them to participate in the labor market (Hernes 1987). This called for developments in the public sector such as home care services, respite care, teaching and counseling.

In many countries, however, the commitment to provide comprehensive public home-care services has been replaced by a concern for the cost of public services (see for example Dahl, this volume). Since the last part of the twentieth century the attention of policy makers has increasingly been centered around the financial burden involved in providing welfare services—rather than questions about how to provide appropriate and good care without placing undue demands on relatives or care workers that was the main focus of much of the feminist literature. In an attempt to contain costs, methods have been developed to ration services such as increasingly detailed rules which dictate service eligibility (Ceci, this volume). This development has led to an infiltration of managerial meanings and understandings in home care which structure the way in which formal care is provided. As Dyck and England (this volume) observe, service workers are told in advance what they are expected to do and they are not allowed to attend to anything unusual that comes up during their visits. Much of the work is prescribed in advance, and work that does not reflect this script simply does not take place or is made invisible.

Here we can observe the tension between those who believe that standardization and rational organization of services will improve quality and efficiency in the social and health care sector (see a further elaboration of this in both Dahl and Olaison, this volume), and those who call for increased flexibility and indeterminacy. This is the point where this book tries to intervene. By re-focusing back on caring but in a new way (Drummond 2004), our aim is to explore notions of good care (a number of authors in this volume re-visit the feminist literature on caring and caregiving including Allen, Dyke and England, and Latimer). We are problematizing the idea that there is a middle ground between universal, standardized knowledge and the ways in which practice is enacted in each situation. Several contributors have drawn on the work of Annemarie Mol (2008) and her associates, who described good care as attentive, meaning paying attention to the particularities of the situation of the people being cared for (both Ceci and Bjornsdottir develop these ideas in relation to home care practice in this volume) where daily life is the starting point for assistance. Knowledge is translated into each situation in such a way that it resonates with the preferences and values of the people. Purkis (this volume) discusses this as the importance of accommodating people's singularities. Mol described good care as creative when workers collectively try out different care arrangements to find the best approach in each situation. This work is embodied and embedded in real life and the aim of practice is improvement.

In Conversation (3)

Davina Allen: I feel like a bit of an interloper in this group, inasmuch as I didn't start off being interested in home care; it's somewhere I ended up as a consequence of an interest in the organization of care, with care conceptualized as work. I guess where I come from is very much from an Everett Hughes kind of position, is to think less about carers and professions, and more about what care is as work, and then look at how it becomes organized and divided up, and the consequences of that. So on a macro level, my thinking is very much informed by the idea that work and other ways that societies choose to organize their work is very much a historical and dynamic process; it changes and evolves in response to a whole range of external influences, technologies, policies, or whatever. It's always moving, it's always interesting, and when it shifts, it has consequences for the workers.

Joanna Latimer: I see care of older people very much as a political site. . . . So I'm very interested in both the organization of care, the distribution, like Davina, of work and care. I don't call it *care*, by the way; I'm very worried about us buying into "This is care," because I don't think it is care; it's delivery, it's provision. I'm not sure when it's care; there may be care, but I don't think we should call it *care* anymore. So I'm very interested in that organizational politics which constructs and works these divisions between the personal, the medical, the social. So social care, what does that mean? You've had a massive stroke, you need a wash: that's social. How can it be social? How is it possibly social? You're sitting there with hemiplegia, you're incontinent, you can't talk, you need a wash—how is that social? How is it even personal?. . .. I think we need to reclaim some space—and we need to reclaim care from its colonization by health services organizations.

Hanne Marlene Dahl: Well, it is a rather large discussion, I think, but I'll start it anyway. I think it's incredibly interesting what you are saying Joanna, about where what is taking place is being labeled as care, or doesn't really qualify as care but what should we label the activity? And have we really thrown the concept of care away? My thinking about this is I think you are very right in diagnosing the problem; we're securing a lot of very critical, normative ideas of good care into what care is, so to speak. So in the sense that we forget that there is this blurring between care and good care, we haven't really been sufficiently attentive to that. So I think we need to develop our analytic concepts much more but does it mean we should throw care away . . . or should we simply make a distinction between "that's care, that's something that's being labeled as care" but *we*, as theorists, think that this is just care, not *good* care. . . . So maybe an alternative solution would that it would be just 'service', borrowing a concept from New Public Management . . . or what would we call it? If you look at it from the outside as a researcher, it's very difficult to say that one or the other way of thinking about care or the ideal of care is better than the other because these cultural-political ideas simply shift from time to time. So I think it's difficult to actually find the position of saying, "well, what then *is* good care?" because that could change culturally, politically but also depending on the personal level . . . it's the voice of the person that really counts because nobody can say in advance what this person would ideally like about care.

Joanna Latimer: We can reclaim it [care]. You see you've got home care, which is a division of labor in welfare states; that's what I was referring to whether it's *home* care or *diabetes* care or *cardiac* care; it's all part of this specialization of services, and they just shove the word *care* on. Care is a mystery when it occurs; it's absolutely mysterious. I wouldn't want to set about saying what it is and how we might recognize it as an it. . . . I think it's reclaiming its opacity, the indirection. We've been living in a culture which asks us all the time to say what things are; well, hang on, we can't. We certainly can't say in advance of an event.

Christine Ceci: But can we say some things in advance? One of the things that Annemarie Mol writes about is the idea that care or good care is not an ideal that can be defined or defended in general terms, that good care is worked out in specific practices. So to use your examples, I think we can say what good cardiac care is, we can say what good diabetes care is; can we say something about what good home care is based on what are the matters of concern of the practices associated with that? So if diabetes care is helping people not to have complications from high blood sugar, then we know we can do some of those things. If home care is about trying to help people live daily life in a way that is more than just endured, then we can maybe say what some of those things might be that would help?

Davina Allen: I'm just wondering if the problem here is about that distinction you are drawing between care and good care, it is about trying to specify ahead what is the good?

Christine Ceci: I don't know that we can say what good care is exactly or specifically, but I think we can say what good care is *like* and what sorts of things would be good. I think that that's probably the most that can be done, and what I would like to try to do is put that into words. So that's really what I've been trying to do in my own paper.

Joanna Latimer: I suppose for me one of the things is the place of care in the life itself, whatever life itself is. And in the life of the people who are doing the care, as well as in the life of the people who are being cared for. It's so easy in this context to think of it as the whole of life; it absorbs everything into it. . . . We were talking earlier about helping people to live a life, a life that is more than just existence . . . but do we know where 'care' is in life for them?

Davina Allen: We don't want to lose sight of how care in the home and care giving is part of a larger picture of how life is managed in contemporary societies.

PRACTICE

Rather than an overarching theoretical orientation, a common analytic strategy and population of interest links the scholarship of the contributors to this book. Interdisciplinary as well as international, contributors were first identified because they tended to use methods of inquiry, such as ethnography, that offer access to the everyday worlds of home care. Each has produced one or more detailed empirical studies of specific aspects of this field and the questions and problems encountered there. Though concerned with differing elements of home care—from analyzing shifts in policy discourse to detailing the specific practices of home care nurses (see Dahl and Björnsdottir respectively, this volume)—their investigations result in clear descriptions of how particular arrangements of home care are working for people and, importantly, analyses of the conditions and policy contexts that are linked to these arrangements.

The orientation to practices is central to this book—home care as such is understood as produced through specific material practices in the context of specific socio-material arrangements. As Moser (2006, 376) argues, "one investigates what something is by asking what it is made to be and how it emerges," an analytical approach linked to Foucault's genealogical method. Several contributors, for example Dahl, Purkis and Ceci (this volume), specifically address the 'conditions of possibility' of current practices, and Purkis in particular uses this framing to speculate about how things might be otherwise. All of the papers developed for this collection illustrate something of *how* home care is currently happening in selected sites—how it is arranged, how it holds together (or not)—and the comparative analysis enabled by gathering these papers together contributes to the development of broader frameworks for thinking through our present concerns.

Though the site of each contributor's research is home care for older people, it is important to recognize that the focus of the analyses are the various social, political and cultural perspectives that organize this site in particular ways—in part this means discerning what is dominant in diverse national contexts and tracing effects in terms of practices. This approach to practices needs to be differentiated from another sense of practices where authors might offer 'how to' guides or prescriptions for practice. Instead our contributors present careful descriptions, and more specifically, display a commitment to interrogating the range of material and discursive practices though which 'home care' is accomplished, with particular attention paid to how questions of knowledge, power and organization are worked out in the realization of care at home for older people. For example Latimer (this volume) asks, what are the practices that establish, and then sustain, a division between the social and the medical?—a question also addressed on an empirical level by Dyck and England (this volume). Ceci (this volume) similarly considers how normalizing practices, such as those that set up human beings as *normally* autonomous and independent, may undermine our capacities to actually help people. These kinds of questions put practices in motion, drawing our attention to how sites are ordered and the ways home care as such may be best thought of as an ongoing and contingent accomplishment (Garfinkel 1967).

In terms of Garfinkel's (1967) ethnomethodology, the objective reality of home care is an ongoing accomplishment of the concerted activities of people—patients, families, formal care providers, administrators, policy makers and so on. What is demonstrated through the careful descriptions of these activities, then, is the constitution of home care. Thus contributors pursue what John Law (1994) describes as a modest sociology, a commitment to analyzing the micro context of care as a means of securing and/or challenging arguments made at the general or macro level. Instead of grand arguments, contributors develop specific analyses grounded in particular contexts that demonstrate the ways that the actualities of everyday life for frail, older people articulate with ideological, political, policy and programmatic discourses. Law (2008) suggests that such modesty in scope and claim helps us to make the problems smaller—or at least more specific. Practices are what we live, or as May (2006, 18) observes following Foucault, "who we are is a matter of our practices." If this is the case, then it is through attention to these—our practices of assisting, accommodating people who are older and perhaps frail—that it may become possible to alter the field of care so that a more responsive practice is possible. As Foucault (1980, 133) observed, "the problem is not changing people's consciousnesses—or what's in their heads—but the political, economic, institutional régime of the production of truth."

In Conversation (4)

Davina Allen: Something to think about for me is whether in fact having a notion of 'what good care is' is very helpful, or whether we need to be turning our attentions to what are the activities, the gestures, or whatever that are necessary in order to enable to people to live at home . . . what are the practices?

Hanne Marlene Dahl: I think we need to develop this term 'practices' a little bit more because you could understand it either in a narrow or broad sense. I think more in the broader sense in terms of institutional practices, not just practices that are relational but rather how these relations—the values, the frames, the interpretations—are related to the larger society, the larger social, cultural, political ideas and discourses.

Anna Olaison: From a communicative perspective, I've studied inter-actions between care managers and the person requesting or requiring care. My focus has been on the micro perspec-tive of institutional practices. What I'm trying to make sense of in my work is how individual solutions are negoti-ated in interactions in the initial assessment meetings, and how they also fit, or are made to fit, the institutional frame-work of home care. Many of the present contradictions are embedded in the present assessment practices when it comes to dilemmas of trying to fit the actual needs of people under the umbrella of a general directive—studying institutional practices at this micro level focuses us on how structures are intertwined and accomplished at this level.

Sirpa Wrede: I've done some work together with Nordic colleagues, and we're trying to understand what has been happening in munici-palities with municipal politicians and officials re-making the whole framework for the policy context and the whole orga-nization of care: what are they actually doing, what are the instruments, what are the politics they are creating in totally remaking the culture of home care . . . how policy becomes practice. . . . And the consequence of all of this for home care as work—when you see how they [care providers] are organiz-ing their behavior in a home in a way that they can live up to the rules they have to live by. So the micro behavior coming to the home is that you don't take off your coat, you don't perhaps even greet the person in a proper way because if you do that then you engage in a social encounter, then things will take longer and you will not meet your schedule. So I think this is how practice gets organized, what gets measured and that's the basis for the fee the client is paying for the service. I'm using the word 'service' here because it's proper in the context of the organization of this work. . . . This type of organization first came to Finland with the international cleaning companies . . . and home care is being organized in the same way, with the same logic. I think this is something that excludes the caring act because it is not on the list. . . . I also think it is a strategy for the people who are doing the actual work to survive. There's not an organization that supports people taking the time, the individual doing the work just consumes her own resources and it makes the difference for the people she is caring for. . . .

Christine Ceci: But what they [care workers] are doing makes perfect sense in the logic of the organization, keeping things running smoothly. It just may not make sense in terms of helping people. . . .

Sirpa Wrede: Because it's not prioritized with the organization, the organization is measuring efficiency, not quality of care. . . .

Mary Ellen Purkis: And I suppose we generate these organizations through the very practices you are describing.

Davina Allen: I see lots of interconnections [in our different work] in that practices in the site of the home are a point of articulation of all those discourses, and power relations—including the division of care or policy or regulations—these are all practices that come to constitute the site.

Joanna Latimer: I think it's time to firm up the ground a bit. I don't know how to do that, but to articulate things in new ways, to give new grounds, new possibilities for people to circulate in their practice, to make moves, to push back certain arrangements of things. . . . And you can push it back and say, "No, it's [home care] this as well." There's always going to be problems with care, whether the funding's insufficient, or resources are poorly distributed; all sorts of issues. So we can't leave it just to the responsibility of those people who, at this time, need help.

NOTES

1. As part of the preparation of this manuscript, the contributors met for two days in April 2009. Prior to our meeting, we exchanged draft papers in order to engage comprehensively and substantively with each other's work. The conversations that ensued were interesting, reflecting our individual and collective effort to do justice to the complexity of the work. Selected excerpts from those conversations are reproduced here with the permission of the participants. These meetings were supported by funding from the Canadian Institutes for Health Research and the Social Sciences and Humanities Research Council.

18   *Christine Ceci, Kristín Björnsdóttir and Mary Ellen Purkis*

REFERENCES

Armstrong, Pat, Hugh Armstrong and Krista Scott-Dixon. 2008. *Critical to care: The invisible women in health services.* Toronto: University of Toronto Press.
Baranek Patricia M., Raisa B. Deber and A. Paul Williams. 2004. *Almost home: Reforming home and community care in Ontario.* Toronto: University of Toronto Press.
Benoit, Cecilia and Helga Halgrimsdottir. 2011. *Valuing care work: Comparative perspectives.* Toronto: University of Toronto Press.
Ceci, Christine, and Mary Ellen Purkis. 2011. Means without ends: justifying supportive home care for frail older people in Canada, 1990–2010. *Sociology of Health and Illness* DOI: 10.111/j.1467-9566.2011.01344x.
Cloyes, Kristin G. 2002. Agonizing care: care ethics, agonistic feminism and political theory of care. *Nursing Inquiry* 9(3): 203–214.
Coles, Romand. 1999. Foucault's dialogical artistic ethos. *Theory, Culture & Society* 8: 99–120.
Cooper, Davina. 2007. "Well, you go there to get off": visiting feminist care ethics through a women's bathhouse. *Feminist Theory* 8(3): 243–262.
Drummond, John. 2004. Nursing and the avant garde. *International Journal of Nursing Studies,* 41: 525–533.
Finch, Janet and Dulcie Groves. Editors. 1983. *A labor of love: Women, work and caring.* London: Routledge and Kegan Paul.
Finlayson, Alan. 2006. "What's the problem?": Political theory, rhetoric and problem-setting. *Critical Review of International Social and Political Philosophy* 9(4), 541–557.
Fisher, Berenice and Joan Tronto. 1990. Towards a feminist theory of caring. In *Circle of care: Work and identity in women's lives,* edited by Emily K. Able and Margaret K. Nelson, 35–62. Albany: State University of New York Press.
Foucault M. 1980. Truth and power. In *Power/Knowledge: Selected interviews and other writings, 1972–1977,* edited by Colin Gordon, 109–133. New York: Pantheon.
Garfinkel, Harold. 1967. *Studies in ethnomethodology.* Englewood Cliffs, NJ: Prentice Hall.
Gilligan, Carol. 1982. *In a different voice: Psychological theory and women's development.* Cambridge, MA: Harvard University Press.
Hernes, Helga Maria. 1987. *Welfare state and women power. Essays in state feminism.* Oslo: Universitetsforlaget.
Holter, Harriet. Editor. 1984. *Patriarchy in a welfare society.* Oslo: Universitatsforlaget.
Law, John. 1994. *Organizing modernity.* Oxford: Blackwell.
——— 2008. On sociology and STS. *The Sociological Review* 56(4): 623–649.
May, Todd. 2006. *The philosophy of Foucault.* Montreal: McGill-Queens University Press.
Mol, Annemarie. 2008. *Logic of Care: Health and the problem of patient choice.* London: Routledge.
Moser, Ingunn. 2006. Disability and the promise of technology. *Information, Communication & Society* 9(3): 373–395.
Watson, Nick, Linda McKie, Bill Hughes, Debra Hopkins, and Sue Gregory. 2004. (Inter)dependence, needs and care: the potential for disability and feminist theorists to develop an emancipatory model. *Sociology* 38(2): 331–350
Waerness, Kari. 2005. Social research, political theory and the ethics of care in a global perspective. In *Dilemmas of care in the Nordic welfare state,* edited by Hanne Marlene Dahl and Tine Erikson, 15–30. London: Ashgate.

Williams, Alison and Valerie A. Crooks. 2008. Introduction: space, place and the geographies of women's caregiving work. *Gender, Place & Culture* 15: 243–247.

Yanzi, Nicole M. and Mark W. Rosenberg. 2008. The contested meanings of home for women caring for children with long-term care needs in Ontario, Canada. *Gender, Place & Culture* 15: 301–315.

Part I
Home

1 Ageing, Independence and Community

Mary Ellen Purkis

What are the conditions of possibility where the frailties of old people would matter? What sort of a world would we inhabit where such frailties could make a difference in decisions that were made about how our lives work and how we would agree that resources ought to be distributed? These questions have formed a foundation from which the ideas presented in this chapter have developed. They were questions raised by Christine Ceci as she planned a meeting of researchers with interests in home-based care for older adults.

I have decided to respond to these questions from a location that takes account of my own and very current personal interests: that is, from a place where I see my parents ageing and hear from them about their daily struggles to make meals interesting, to maintain a sense of social inclusion having retired and moved away from a community in which they were active and well known, and the considerations involved in letting go of household tasks that they have been able to do, and have often taken pride in doing, for an entire lifetime together—but in which they no longer have any interest and with which their bodies are not really willing to engage anymore.

Against these personal observations and the questions that have prompted them, the chapter is also shaped by critical readings of the concepts of home and community. I have chosen to focus these readings on the writings of novelist Marilynne Robinson, specifically her award-winning novel *Gilead* (2004) and the critical commentary on community of Giorgio Agamben as set out in his challenging text, *The Coming Community* (1993). Other contemporary academic literature is used to draw out meanings from these core texts.

My intention here is to investigate the possibilities of ageing in contemporary western communities, acknowledging up front the necessity and the danger of over-generalizing the characteristics, limitations and possibilities inherent in such communities, and the limits of choosing to live in such communities within a societal value system that prizes independence. Perhaps at its core my question is this: as elders age and become more frail, what sorts of accommodations can be made to their locations in community to enhance opportunities for independent living?

AN ALL-TOO-COMMON STORY . . .

My parents moved from our family home in an urban center located on the edge of the Canadian prairies to live closer to where I currently live on the west coast of Canada. I feel myself frequently called upon to generate occasions that remind us all of the long-gone days of a busy and active family engaged in our home community. I continue to be active in my own community—but my community is not their community. I have to step out of my community (of work and friends) in order to step into theirs (as a daughter, sister, aunt) and there is very little overlap between these two communities. As things currently stand, I do not mind the movement between these two communities and indeed, the different pace of the two communities creates some perspective for me as I make choices about how I live my life. And so, to some extent at least, I do accommodate their frailties as I seek to adjust the pace of my life when I join in community with them. Their frailties do make a difference to me as I live my life and I make changes in the pace and direction of my life as I take account of those differences.

How realistic is it to imagine that such accommodations could be mass-produced?

As I think about my own situation, I acknowledge that I have not married and have no children, and I can easily place myself in my parents' shoes and wonder, how will I be cared for as I age? I look around me in a city to which many older people migrate for their later years because the climate is so considerate—and I see many different arrangements that people may choose (but I use that word very cautiously) to answer that question for themselves: choices that often seem not quite as considerate as the climate.

In this city ageing people may choose to remain in a home that they either own or rent. Over time, they may need to supplement that home with material and personnel supports that enable them to maintain their independence in their own home. But, with economic times being more challenging now than at anytime since these elders may have been children themselves, I wonder how many of them worry about their ability to sustain themselves in these so-called independent situations through to the end of their lives.

For those feeling less than secure about living independently, they may choose to live in one of many communal arrangements available. While more intentional arrangements are described in the ageing literature (for example, Askham, Briggs, Norman and Redfern 2007; Malmberg 1999; Mitchell 1999; Thomas and Blanchard 2009), anonymous institutional players such as provincial health authorities, for-profit housing corporations, not-for-profit housing collectives or faith communities most often operate these communal living spaces. Where individuals themselves can organize them, living arrangements can be created that mean older adults may have the advantage of collective living (sharing costs associated with home ownership, in-home care provision, food and a sense of social inclusion) with some vestiges of independence.

Still others may have minimal choices. 'The authorities'—whether physicians, case managers or relatives—may take those choices away from them 'for their own safety'. Here, the sorts of housing options available seem very narrow—mostly taking the shape of institutions that, try as they might, cannot transcend their historical compulsion to aggregate people for the purposes of providing cost-effective custodial care. And in case I seem to be valorizing the home too much and associating it with independence, research demonstrates that institution-like custodial care is also easily achieved within a home setting.

A THEORETICAL APPROACH

In seeking to come to grips with the conditions of possibility—those features of everyday life that could support a full engagement in life—for accommodating the myriad unique needs and desires of older adults as they seek options for living independently in the community, I have been drawn to the work of Giorgio Agamben and in particular his text *The Coming Community* (1993). There are two key attractions to Agamben's work on community: first, his approach to the idea of community is radical and presents a strong challenge to an uncritical portrayal of community as welcoming and supportive; and second, he offers an interesting way of thinking about the politics of community. In the explorations that follow, I will present a reading of Agamben's thought in relation to the central concern regarding the conditions of possibility whereby the frailties of older adults would matter.

In *The Coming Community*, Agamben considers the possibility of a community that does not rely on a claim of identity. Taking as his exemplar the activities of Chinese students at the time of the Tiananmen Square uprising, he notes that what was striking about that event was the response from the Chinese State in relation to the "relative absence of determinate contents of their [the students'] demands" (84). Agamben reminds us of two 'demands' made by the students: first, democracy and freedom, "notions too generic and broadly defined to constitute the real object of a conflict," and second, "the rehabilitation of Hu Yao-Bang," a demand that had already been met before the deaths at Tiananmen Square had occurred (84). So what, asks Agamben, can account for the extreme response from the Chinese government in response to the refusal of the students to cease their quiet, peaceful but very public protests?

Making a deliberate link between the constitution of community and the effects of politics, Agamben's argument is that "the novelty of the coming politics is that it will no longer be a struggle for the conquest or control of the State, but a struggle between the State and the non-State (humanity), an insurmountable disjunction between whatever singularity and the State organization" (84). Agamben's text presages a new ground for political struggles. Drawing on the dramatic events in Tiananmen Square for an exemplar of this new ground, he draws our attention to the underlying facts of the matter: this was no pure political struggle between identifiable political parties. While the students could be said to form an identifiable community of sorts, their demands, as a group, were both too broad (democracy) to be addressed (or even rejected) in any sort of obvious way and also lacking substance (their hero, Hu Yao-Bang, had already been rehabilitated before the protests had begun). What then can account for the Chinese state's extreme response? Agamben's answer is that, as an exemplar of the coming politics, it was simply (and, of course, not so simply) the presence of the students in a public place acting in a way "such as it always matters" (1). Agamben's argument is that the students did not need a unifying, identifying narrative to provoke the response from the Chinese state. Their presence in the Square, expressing their broad *and* specific concerns seemed to be a sufficient reason for the government to take action.

It strikes me that my concerns about the options for living independently in contemporary communities can be addressed through reference to Agamben's ideas—largely because of this approach to the political. My personal concerns about my parents and myself bear, in all likelihood, some similarity to the concerns of the older people living in my immediate community as well as in similar communities across Canada and much of the western world. Having said this, our *particular* concerns may well be quite different from one another—as the range of housing 'options' suggests. Not only is it *unlikely* that we would ever find the political motivation to join together 'in community' in our efforts to demand the creation of innovative living spaces that respond to our particular needs or the 'whatever singularities' (as Agamben calls them) but also, as for the students in Tiananmen Square, it is *unnecessary* if what we are seeking is to provoke a response from those who currently plan, fund and operate those spaces.

In order to comprehend the implications of Agamben's approach to politics, the concept of "*whatever* singularities" deserves some further consideration.

Whatever Singularities

Agamben begins his treatise on community by giving consideration to the individuals who constitute the coming community. Ironically, in order to give consideration to the future, he turns to ancient philosophy and draws on the Scholastic enumeration of the transcendentals—the goods that cut across time and contexts and speak to the quality of relationships that one might expect to arise from community. But rather than focusing on those goods, for example "whatever entity is one, true, good, or perfect" (1), he focuses instead on the adjective that conditions all those goods: *whatever.*

Acknowledging the common and current translation of that word as meaning indifference (one is reminded here of the common parlance of adolescents today who use the word in just that way), he reinstates the Latin meaning, which is to say that 'whatever' (*quodlibet*) is "being such that it always matters" (1). And he reminds us that in the Latin, whatever "always already contains . . . a reference to the will (*libet*). Whatever being has an original relation to desire" (1). Agamben then argues that

> the Whatever in question here relates to singularity not in its indifference with respect to a common property (to a concept, for example: being red, being French, being Muslim), but only in its being *such as it is*. Singularity is thus freed from the false dilemma that obliges knowledge to choose between the ineffability of the individual and the intelligibility of the universal. . . . In this conception, such-and-such being is reclaimed from its having this or that property, which identifies it as belonging to this or that set, to this or that class (the reds, the French, the Muslims)—and it is reclaimed not for another class nor for the simple generic absence of any belonging, but for its being-*such*, for belonging itself. (Agamben, 1–2, emphasis in original)

My reading of Agamben here is that age, for instance, is a very blunt tool of identification for determining community. Programs of home support or programs of care delivered through institutions that are calculated by the state as 'affordable' ways of reducing the higher costs associated with caring for older adults in acute care institutions are much less accommodating to the needs of those requiring additional support if such programs are only available to individuals 80 years and older. In creating such programs, we generate a kind of community that is indifferent to the singularities of an older adult, *such as she is*. We might similarly argue that 'ability' is another such blunt tool that is often invoked in order to move people out of independent situations in community and into collective communities that are, for the most part, incapable of supporting independence.

In contrast to the institutional—and political—response to care for ageing adults characterized by the development of arbitrary programs of home-based support, I am reminded of some recent interactions I have had with a women's religious community that has established a care home for their ageing members. The care home is located on the third floor of the residence where many of these religious women have spent the better part of their adult lives living together in a highly identity-based community. However, within the context of providing nursing care for those members who are ageing and becoming increasingly frail, the matron described to me the many unique "accommodations" that are made for those living in the extended care wing of the Mother House, accommodations that appear to respond to the *'whatever* singularities' of these members. For one sister, the door to the en suite bathroom had been removed and a curtain installed instead because she most often mobilized by using her wheelchair and found accessing the bathroom difficult when the door was in place as it was in all other rooms. For another sister, a small table was installed in the bay window to enable her to continue to use her sewing machine, with the advantage of full sunlight from the window in her room. This table was installed in such a way that it was sufficiently robust to support the sewing machine—but could be easily removed without a trace when another resident might subsequently occupy the room.

Another instance that fills out the meaning of both the way I wish to use the word accommodation here as well as Agamben's use of the notion of the '*whatever* singularity' comes from a passage of the Pulitzer prize-winning novel *Gilead*, written by Marilynne Robinson. In this passage, John Ames, the narrator of the story, is sharing an experience of walking through his town to the church where he is minister to his parishioners:

> The light in the room was beautiful this morning, as it often is. It's a plain old church and it could use a coat of paint. But in the dark times I used to walk over before sunrise just to sit there and watch the light come into that room. *I don't know how beautiful it might seem to any-one else.* I felt much at peace those mornings, praying over very dreadful things sometimes—the Depression, the wars . . . In those days as I have said, I might spend most of a night reading. Then, if I woke up still in my armchair, and if the clock said four or five, I'd think how pleasant it was to walk through the streets in the dark and let myself into the church and watch dawn come in the sanctuary. I loved the sound of the latch lifting. The building has settled into itself so that when you walk down the aisle, you can hear it yielding to the burden of your weight. It's a pleasanter sound than an echo would be, *an obliging, accommodating sound. You have to be there alone to hear it.* (Robinson, 70, emphasis added).

This passage represents a paradox of community and accommodation. John Ames is an elderly minister, residing in the fictional town of Gilead, Iowa. He was married as a young man and had a daughter with his first wife but both the daughter and the wife died when he was still quite young and, for many years afterwards, he remained a widower. In the preceding passage Reverend Ames acknowledges that it might only be him who experiences watching the sun rise from inside the church as beautiful. He is alone, yet he is in a space that only a collective—a community—could create: a church. As a building it connotes a collective space for worship. Anyone can establish an altar at which private worship can be engaged in as his or her own personal space. However, his weight is accommodated within this communal space—but you have to be alone in this space to hear it!

In this passage Robinson uses the word "accommodating" to refer to the sound of the church building that accepts the unique weight—including the unique burdens—of the man who enters the sanctuary to witness the sunrise alone. The passage lends meaning to the idea of accommodation as I hear it being used by the matron of the extended care unit—it is a singular act—"you have to be there alone to hear it." Similarly, the accommodations made by the matron are singular acts made by staff in the extended care unit in relation to the *whatever* singularities of the ageing sisters. Just as the sound of the church accommodating the burdens of Reverend Ames in *Gilead* can only be heard when he is there alone, just so the accommodations made for individual sisters are made for them alone and may have meaning for them alone—although something of that meaning is shared by the matron who oversees the work or action required to accommodate the needs of the elder sisters. The same 'accommodation' could not be made for all those residing in the extended care unit. They may not experience it as an accommodation to *their* needs but rather the institution of a rule—in all likelihood for the benefit of staff. In contrast to those institutionalized practices that we all seem to know too well, the way that the matron makes changes to a room occupied by a specific sister in order to accommodate her changing health and personal needs, the frailties of these particular old people are made to matter. What are the conditions of possibility for such care?

CROSSING THE THRESHOLD: THE FACE OF AGEING

To answer this question, I return again to Robinson's novel. The novel is written in the form of a letter. As an older man, John Ames re-marries, to a young woman with whom he has a son. As he nears the end of his life, he is writing of his life in Gilead as a letter to his young son, a letter that he intends to be read by the son long after Ames' death. He is writing about the singularities of his life and hopes in this way to share something of that life with his son when his son will be old enough, and perhaps curious enough about his father, to want to understand him better than Ames imagines he is able to now while he is just a boy of five or six years of age.

Ames writes about his early life and the time when his daughter, Rebecca, was born:

> While I was holding her, she opened her eyes. I know she didn't really study my face. Memory can make a thing seem to have been much more than it was. But I know she did look right into my eyes. And I'm glad I knew it at the time, because now, in my present situation, now that I am about to leave this world, I realize there is nothing more astonishing than a human face . . . you feel your obligation to a child when you have seen it and held it. *Any human face is a claim on you,*

because you can't help but understand the singularity of it, the courage and loneliness of it. (Robinson, 66, emphasis added)

Robinson's text draws out a condition of the sort of care that the matron has instituted for sisters living in the extended care unit. The matron describes her work in that context as though she responds to the claim the sisters have on her. Agamben writes of this radical relationship in this way:

Whatever adds to singularity only an emptiness, only a threshold: Whatever is a singularity plus an empty space, a singularity that is *finite* and, nonetheless, indeterminable according to a concept. But a singularity plus an empty space can only be a pure exteriority, a pure exposure. *Whatever, in this sense, is the event of an outside* (. . .) It is important here that the notion of the "outside" is expressed in many European languages by a word that means "at the door" (*fores* in Latin is the door of the house, *thyrathen* in Greek literally means "at the threshold"). The *outside* is not another space that resides beyond a determinate space, but rather, it is the passage, the exteriority that gives it access—in a word, it is its face, its *eidos* (Agamben, 66–67).

There is something interesting here that points back to a romantic ideal of community, invoked perhaps when we seek to dispense with the call that elders have on 'us'. We claim that while they live 'in community' they will somehow be cared for within that community. But they live behind doors that render their lives all but invisible—until some event occurs: a fall, a severe illness that requires hospitalization, a determination that they are no longer safe. They can then be removed from 'the community', or at least their independence in living in that community can be significantly curtailed. Institutionalized forms of care are placed around them or they are placed within institutions of care.

But these spaces they occupy when they are living independently are interesting: they are private—exclusive—independent—when 'we' wish them to be. We can invoke elders' 'right' to privacy, but just up to a point. Then 'we' can invade that space and, making it public, we can then exclude them to the institutional life of residential care—the camp. According to Agamben, the camp is the space opened when the exception becomes the rule or the normal situation, as was the case in Germany in the period immediately before and throughout World War II. And here is a location to give consideration to the politics of caring for frail elders. When their interests in living independently can so easily be set aside by those of us who are family members or members of caring professions or members of local governments and health authorities in the name of 'safety' or 'responsibility', how different is that form of violence from that imposed on the students in Tiananmen Square and during the 1930s and 1940s in Germany?

There is an important contrast in the matron's (political) actions of accommodating the *whatever* singularities of the ageing sisters to those of us who would institutionalize care for the frail elderly. She is acknowledging that the sisters have particular and different interests from one another. And in seeking to accommodate an ageing sister, the matron takes account of her *being such as it is*. In Agamben's world, this is not an accommodation directed toward this or that particular property of the other but neither does it disregard those properties in favour of an "insipid generality" (Agamben, 2) that might be called 'patient focused care'. Imagine the powerful authority of a care provider who can make such accommodations in the face of institutionalizing trends to the contrary: she appears to respond to the face of the ageing sister, accepting the claim it has on her. And, as such, she accomplishes the notion of "threshold" advanced by Agamben:

> Whatever adds to singularity only an emptiness, only a threshold: Whatever is a singularity plus an empty space, a singularity that is finite and, nonetheless, indeterminable (. . .) Whatever, in this sense, is the event of an outside (. . .) The outside is not another space that resides beyond a determinate space, but rather, it is the passage, the exteriority that gives it access—in a word, it is its face, its *eidos*. (Agamben, 66–67)

In being claimed by the face of the other, the matron accommodates the *whatever* singularities of the sister, occupying the space that is neither interior to the sister (she does not need to *know* with any certainty what the sister wants/needs) nor exterior (she resists instituting the change elsewhere in the extended care unit as an instance of 'care for elders'). I want to conclude this chapter by focusing on the politics of Agamben's thought—to argue that such actions as I have theorized here and represented by the precise and unique practices of the matron are instances of actions conditioned by what Agamben would call the coming politics.

THE POLITICS OF ACCOMMODATING OLDER ADULTS

The threshold added to the *whatever* singularity of each elder facing a care provider who holds, in his or her hands, access to a quotient of care (e.g., specified hours of home support time, access to a physiotherapist, a financial subsidy to offset some part of the cost of a long-term care facility)—is a threshold that is "only an emptiness . . . an empty space . . . the passage, the exteriority that gives it access . . . it is its face" (Agamben, 67).

I need to contrast the careful accommodations made by the matron to the reaction of an agent of institutionalizing community supports in the very same municipality—that is, the reaction of a case manager to the living circumstances of my parents. Both now in their 80s, my mother is living with dementia and my father is her primary caregiver. Having recognized significant cognitive decline in my mother's ability to report on her own health, her general practitioner referred my mother to the Geriatric Assessment Unit operated by the regional health authority. Based at one of the large hospitals in town, members of that service then linked us into the associated community support agency and, as part of that mechanism, we had a visit from a case manager, a health care professional responsible for monitoring the ability of older adults to live independently in the community. Upon entering my parents' home, the case manager immediately 'summed up' their circumstances, declaring their home 'unsafe'—largely because of the stairs that are necessary to move from the garage to the kitchen and, from there, additional stairs to access the bedrooms and bathrooms, which are located on the top floor of a three storey townhouse. At no time during his visit to my parents' home did he seek to test out his statement regarding the safety of the living space my parents occupy.

Here we confront an instance of the state's intervention into the business of 'caring' for the old and frail. As such we have stepped into the deconstructed terrain that Agamben claims has previously firmed up politico-philosophical foundations. Agamben, turning back to Aristotle for the distinction, shows how the notion of politics was reserved for those aspects of life dealing with activities beyond the (privacy of the) family home:

> Human beings began living in families, then they acquired slaves and formed villages, until finally they achieved a self-sufficient mode of life. But to treat this as nothing more than a history is to misunderstand the nature of the boundary that human beings cross when their community becomes self-sufficient, and to assume . . . that political life can be simply added on to human life. Aristotle, however, expressly denies this . . . to be truly human one must be a member of a polis, for it is only as such that one can truly speak. (Norris 2000, 40)

Politics, for Agamben, "occupies the threshold on which the relation between the living being and the logos is realized. In the 'politicization' of bare life—the metaphysical task par excellence—the humanity of living man is decided" (Agamben 1998, 8). And so, while we may have been lured into thinking, as young adults, that the home is a place of refuge from the politics of administering human life, growing old and frail forces us to confront that this is no longer the case—and may never have been in any case. This is the politico-philosophical foundation that Agamben disrupts in his writing.

In taking up this admittedly dismal assessment of the possibilities for action and resistance in the domain of everyday life, I return again to the increasingly remarkable and courageous actions of the matron. In her actions, I would like to advance the claim that resistance to the organizing effects of institutional care regimes is possible—but not easy—to achieve.

FRAGILE COMPROMISES AND MODEST
ACCOUNTS OF RESISTANCE

The first act of resistance that can be detected in the matron's actions is that rather than dampening down the need for their living space to be adjusted, the matron moves into that space to find opportunities for accommodation. It would appear that having been claimed by the faces of the ageing sisters, she responds to that claim by seeking accommodations that respond to the *whatever* singularities of the sisters. It could be argued that a key difference between the situation of the matron's response to the sisters and that of the case manager to my parents is that the matron is working with ageing women whose frailties have been fairly well described and therefore she has a wealth of knowledge to draw from in developing responses to their evolving frailties, whereas the case manager enters my parents home for the first time, has not previously met them, has no prior knowledge of their capacities and weaknesses.

But recall the previous discussion of the threshold: in occupying that space that is neither interior nor exterior, such knowledge of the person is unnecessary (which is not the same thing as saying that such knowledge is not useful in many respects). Rather, actions undertaken within the threshold seek only to keep both the interior and exterior in play—and as such represent potentially fleeting opportunities that might be described as fragile compromises in the resolution of disputes.

These decisions that we all face—about how to live our lives, about how much risk we are willing to incorporate into our everyday practices of living 'independently' in our chosen place—are ultimately disputable and clearly, when the case manager came to visit my parents, despite their efforts to present themselves as effective, able individuals, he read them as living dangerously and perhaps unnecessarily so—underlining their (in) ability to think about their circumstances properly.

A fragile compromise might have emerged had the case manager asked how my parents use their chosen place, how my mother uses both hands on the handrail to draw herself upward from the kitchen to her bedroom, how swiftly she still negotiates those steps—and how, admittedly after a fall, my father supported her body against his as they negotiated the steps together to get from one floor to the other. At the time during which she was recovering from her fall, she moved much less swiftly and with considerably more pain—but she did not complain about the pain. She was willing to be subjected to it to be in her home and to move about in that home in a way that expresses her "being such that it always matters" (Agamben, 1).

Disregarding the case manager's advice comes, no doubt, with some risks itself. But his obligation to fulfill the state requirement of an institutionalized form of care for older adults can likely be counted on to ensure his regular return to check in on my parents. Setting aside the advice to move to a one-level home is not easy for my parents. And it brings with it a whole series of questions about doing the 'right thing'. But it also represents just one (small) moment of resistance that over the next few years will no doubt be forgotten in the myriad other moments of resistance they will engage as they seek to occupy the threshold of independence as they age. This is a challenging space to occupy. It is neither right nor wrong to be there. Its location cannot be determined—one simply *is* there at those moments of resistance when the *whatever* singularities are called into question by the effects of institutionalizing practice.

The matron's actions suggest that with experience and knowledge of how elders live in their places, one might positively engage the *whatever* singularities to make the frailties of older people matter—at least within the confines of prescribed home. While it may seem little and even insufficient to some, in contrast to the violence of exclusion that many older adults experience, those accommodations mark important opportunities to practice humanely.

REFERENCES

Agamben, Giorgio. 1993. *The coming community.* Translated by Michael Hardt. Edited by Sandra Buckley, Michael Hardt and Brian Massumi, Theory out of Bounds. Minneapolis: University of Minnesota Press.

Agamben, Giorgio. 1998. *Homo Sacer: Sovereign power and bare life.* Translated by Daniel Heller-Roazen. Stanford, CA: Stanford University Press.

Askham, Janet, Kate Briggs, Ian Norman and Sally Redfern. 2007. Care at home for people with dementia: as in a total institution? *Ageing and Society* 27: 3–24.

Malmberg, Bo. 1999. Swedish group homes for people with dementia. *Generations* 23(3): 82–84.

Mitchell, Rosas. 1999. Home from home: a model of daycare for people with dementia. *Generations* 23(3): 78–81.

Norris, Andrew. 2000. Giorgio Agamben and the politics of the living dead. *Diacritics* 30(4): 38–58.

Robinson, Marilynne. 2004. *Gilead.* New York: Farrar, Straus and Giroux.

Thomas, William H., and Janice M. Blanchard. 2009. Moving beyond place: ageing in community. *Generations* 33(2): 12–17.

2 Home Care and Frail Older People
Relational Extension and the Art of Dwelling

Joanna Latimer

Nothing comes without its world.

—Donna Haraway 1997, 37

This paper is exploratory and mainly discursive. Drawing on a number of sources, it explores home and care in terms of relational extension, keeping and the art of dwelling.

Care in relation to older people has increasingly been constituted in terms of provision and service-user/service-provider dyads. To get care-as-provision there has to be a construction of need through the gaze of medicine, nursing and social work. Care-as-provision not only constitutes the ageing body as increasingly in deficit, but can extrude other ways of understanding. Despite in many ways appearing to be private, enacted behind closed doors, seemingly "backstage" (Goffman 1959, 1966), spaces of care are inscribed by discourses of care-as-provision and risk. The home as a space of provision and risk entails "bodywork" (Twigg 2000a, 2000b) and increasing surveillance through assistive technology (Disabled Living Foundation 2008). But home and care are sites of performance and identity-work, for both cared-for and carers.

This space of identity-work has to be understood in terms of dominant cultural preoccupations including the body *and the home* as sites of enhancement, aesthetics and consumption (Featherstone 1982; Hurdley 2006; Miller 2001; Wiles 2005), youthfulness (Tulle 2008), auto-mobility (Latimer and Munro 2006) and self-determination, autonomy, enterprise and activity (Strathern, 1992), possession and lifestyle choice (Bauman 2003, Skeggs 2004), each of which are valued as the marks of the healthy, responsible 'good' citizen (Hillman 2008). Like the bedside in hospitals, the space of home and care can thus be understood as a "complex location" (Latimer 2000, drawing on Cooper).

Critically, in the UK at least, there is a "constituting of classes" (Latimer 1997, 2000) of work, people and things in which care of the elderly, home care and care home work is denigrated and denigrating. The work is low paid, frequently part-time, and like the very frail and the aged themselves, potentially stigmatizing (Goffman 1963). In the UK, the everyday work of care has been divided off from the everyday work of medical intervention (Latimer 2009c), with qualified nurses and social workers managing and coordinating delivery of care packages, rather than being directly involved in care work themselves. Many older people are now cared for directly by migrant workers (Doyle and Timonen 2009), who are themselves also positioned, by their very mobility and absence of roots, as "precarious labour" (Papadopoulos, Stephenson, and Tsianos 2008). One of the problems is that this kind of work is constituted as semi-skilled, maintenance work: it, and the people being cared for, the frail elderly, are figured as having no future, no "prospects ahead of them" (Latimer 2000), they are going nowhere, either in terms of their health or in terms of their (social) mobility. In addition, the frail elderly are easily figured as losing their distinctive identity as "possessive individuals" (Skeggs 2004) and as being in a process of withdrawal, literally shrinking in terms of corporeal presence, including relinquishing their possessions as they downsize, and, with them, expectations and identity. As Cohen (1994, drawing on Myerhoff 1978) elaborates, older people can so easily seem to lose definition and become invisible, inchoate (Latimer 1999).

This figuring of the frail elderly, and the work around supporting them at home, constructs their bodies and them as failing and as "unknowing" (Latimer 2009b). I want to call this the *deficit model* (Latimer 2010) of older people and of their care. Seeing the body and the older person as in deficit is, of course, the effect of a particular perspective, one that, as will be seen, has pervasive effects, including making us blind to the affective, processual and relational dimensions of care.

While not wishing to undermine the suffering and pain sometimes involved, I do want to stress that this figuring of the elderly frail as in deficit ignores the relational dimension of helplessness and frailty. If we shift perspective for a moment, we can see how helplessness and frailty do not simply inhere in certain bodies, but are an effect of an interaction between certain kinds of bodies and their cultural and social worlds. For example, people with so-called dementia find themselves in social worlds that they do not fit (Schillmeier 2009), and this lack of fit between how they are, their body and the world means that they find themselves as 'out of line' (Munro and Belova 2009), all of which does not just intensify the experience and the condition (Schofield 2008) but partly constructs the condition itself (see also Kraeftner and Kröell 2009).

So what is required is the possibility of shifting perspectives and a way to refigure the figure of the frail elderly, and therefore the people that work with them, differently. [1] Questions arise as to how we can bring into view methods, narratives and discourses that circulate difference in ways that help deconstruct these old hierarchies: ways of imagining that revalue both the aged and the frail [2] and the care that some older people require. I am thinking here of May and Flemming's (1997) paper in which they stress the importance of imagining ways of caring that are distinct from those rooted through main stream medicine. There has been an emerging emphasis in social policy on exploring ways of thinking of the home as a 'space' of care and of 'care in place'. These new approaches privilege attention to the meaning of home and issues of self-determination, dignity, individuality, privacy and choice and have been groundbreaking. But as I suggest in what follows, these discourses, as important as they are, circulate a stress on home and care as connected to individual identity, and the maintenance of place and presentation of self, or 'face' (Goffman 1955, 1966). What the emphasis on individuality, place and face does not address is how care is not an add-on to people's lives and worlds, something simply provided to support a life in a home, but processual, relational and, critically, world-forming.

The starting point then, for re-imagining could be to posit a different, less-functional notion of care and the involvement of practitioners and older people as embodied persons in relations (e.g., Rudge 2009; Savage 1995). In what follows, I extend this focus through drawing together Strathern's theory of relational extension (1988, 1991, 1993, 1997) with Martin Heidegger's (1978) theory of dwelling to offer a way to re-imagine spaces of home-care that focuses on care as relational and the materiality of home and care as *Mitsein* (or being-with) (Heidegger 1962).

Specifically, I stress embodiment and relational extension, and forms of organization embedded in a view of care routed in "body-world relations" (Latimer 2009a). Here I explore how by bringing being-with alongside being-in-the world (*Dasein*) (Heidegger 1962), we can think of home and care in terms of locale, materiality and relationality rather than just in terms of individualization, place, autonomy, choice and self. That is, I return to an idea of a space of care and dwelling in terms of locale (Heidegger 1978), rather than in terms of face and place. I draw on an exegesis of a famous poem by Philip Larkin, *Mr Bleaney* written with Rolland Munro (Latimer and Munro 2009).[3] While this exegesis is rather cumbersome, in the current context I use it to illustrate the art of dwelling in terms of how routines and habits, and what we keep, are important, but how their importance does not just come from their being personal or functional, matters of autonomous choice, but as critical to the making up of home and a space of care as *Mitsein*, or being-with (Heidegger 1962). I then illustrate the mysterious space of care and its possibility for dwelling and the making and unmaking of worlds together, through a brief excerpt from the film *The Diving Bell and the Butterfly*. I analyze this excerpt for how it helps illustrate care and the art of dwelling in terms of *Mitsein* and affect, and how what is kept can turn us over as well as decide our lives. I end with the five cats of *Akropolis*, a community for older people in the Netherlands, organized in ways that stress the art of living and the engagement of older people in world-forming, no matter how frail (see also Bendien 2010, Becker 2008). In this space care is as much about making a life and being-with as it is about provision in the fulfillment of needs, however individuated, because this only re-routes care back to existence through face, self and choice.

THE SCALE OF THE ISSUE

This book addresses issues that arise from shifts in health care organization that seem to mean that people, particularly the chronically sick, disabled and the elderly, are increasingly receiving care at home or in a care home, rather than in hospital, and that responsibility for provision is increasingly divided between different services, the private sector and the family. Budlender (2008) has also investigated how this effect works across many nation states.

Health and social policy since 1990 in the UK, for example, has put more and more emphasis on older people and people with severe, disabling illness staying in the community sector, either at home or in a home. In a sense this shift represents a reversal of Foucault's observation of the hospital as a site for the medicalization of illness, so that what we are witnessing in some way is medicine's abandonment, or the demedicalization, of the chronically sick, the disabled and the frail and a concomitant institutionalization and medicalization of the home.

Home care can be needed when people live in their 'own' homes or in a residential home. In 2004, an estimated 410,000 older people lived in residential and nursing homes across the UK (OFT 2005). In 2008, there were estimated to be about 394,000 older people out a total of 418,000 people in residential care (Help the Aged 2009), of whom 182,000 were supported by community care. There are about 15,700 private, voluntary and Local Authority care homes in the UK providing care at an estimated annual value of more than £8 billion per annum (OFT 2005). Large numbers of people are also noted as in need of care and support at home. A survey carried out in 2005 by the NHS Information Centre showed that an astonishing 98,200 households (28% of households) received intensive home care in 2005 (defined as more than 10 contact hours and 6 or more visits during the week). This represents a 6% increase from the 2004 figure of 92,300 (NHS Information Centre 2006).

Of course, this represents only a fraction of 'care' provided: family, particularly women and increasingly children, carry what is thought of as the burden of care, with an estimated 4,900,000 people giving care to older people in England in 2004 (Audit Commission 2004). 2.8 million people aged 50 and over provide unpaid care and 5% of people aged 85+ provide unpaid care, with carers, who are mainly female, currently saving the UK economy an estimated £87 billion a year (Help the Aged 2009).

The historical and political basis of an increasing need for homecare is complex (Budlender 2008). Resources here are limited and there has been an increasing shift toward the use of private organizations. In the UK as elsewhere, there have been difficulties over regulation of residential and nursing home care of the elderly and chronic sick, with more and more of this care being privatized and contracted out to charities and other independently run organizations (Audit Commission 2004). Similarly, home care, the care of a person in their 'own' home by nurses and other paid carers, can also be contracted out to private organizations. A parallel effect, particularly in the context of the intensification of a sense of the risks of being at home on your own when you are old or disabled, is the development of assistive technology, such as telecare services, that supposedly allows people to stay at home but that provides remote monitoring and surveillance (Lopez and Domenech 2009). [4] In England and Wales (but not Scotland), people are means tested and their needs differentiated between personal and nursing or medical needs, the former being paid for by the individual, the latter being provided at no extra cost by the NHS and/or local authority.

The quality of care and life of residents in residential and nursing homes varies enormously. A recent report by the Commission for Social Care Inspection (2008) in England suggests that around a third of all care homes for older people are rated as 'poor' or 'adequate' by government inspectors and that 22% of older people assisted by their councils are being placed in such homes. Furthermore,

> being rated as poor or adequate means that such homes are likely to have failed to meet a number of the national minimum standards which inspectors check against when visiting homes. Characteristically, such homes may have fewer staff and as a consequence residents wait longer for such basic needs as food and drink to be met, or assistance to use the toilet. (The Relatives and Residents Association, 2009)

While for many a residential or nursing home offers subsistence, hotel services, basic nursing and medical intervention (if you are lucky), questions arise as to whether or not they offer much of a life. For example, BBC Radio 4's *Today* program (June 4, 2008) recently reported on an investigation of life in care homes based on covert participation by Deddie Davies, a "sprightly 70 year old" and trustee of *Compassion in Care*, who was determined to give the elderly a voice. Deddie compiled an audio report on her experience and observations on being admitted to a home, much of which was recorded in situ. She states that care home life was like "slow death." What the report shows is an extraordinary level of inactivity and loneliness, with minimal interaction, between residents or between residents and staff. Critically, while there is provision of a clean and safe environment, meals and basic care, the overall impression of the life in the home that Deddie gives is that people are, in a sense, stabled; they are "just waiting," filling in time, eking out an existence. Deddie points out how she is not particularly frail and that "it's not until you put yourself into the position of utter helplessness that you realize how much more is needed to make the days worthwhile other than being washed and fed."

My suggestion is that this kind of helplessness is not just a condition that inheres in the frail, because of poor mobility, sight, speech, hearing, health and so on and so forth. Helplessness is, as Deddie helps us to see, *relational*: it is as much a construction of the interaction of body-persons and their environments, or as I have designated it, body-world relations (Latimer 2009a).

It is assumed that people would prefer to remain at home (OFT 2005). Care provision for people in their home should redress some of the imbalances of power associated with situations like that described by Deddie, because of the supposed relationship between ownership, control, independence and autonomy. However, Twigg (2000a, 2000b) in her work on home care and the 'social' bath, has shown the quality of life of people living in their own homes who require intense care also varies enormously. A home can become increasingly institutionalized: de-privatized, colonized, with the institution of similar processes of objectification as are to be found in care homes. She emphasizes the complexity of community care, and how it is accomplished, as deeply implicated in the ordinary and mundane routines and habits that support a life. Gott et al. (2004), in their investigation of people's attitudes toward dying at home, also illuminate great complexity here:

> Participants identified that home was more than a physical location, representing familiarity, comfort and the presence of loved ones. While participants anticipated that home would be their ideal place of care during dying, practical and moral problems associated with it were recognised by many. Some had no informal carer. Others did not want to be a 'burden' to family and friends, or were worried about these witnessing their suffering. Those who had children did not wish them to deliver care that was unduly intimate. Concerns were expressed about the quality of care that could be delivered at home, particularly in relation to accommodating health technologies and providing adequate symptom relief. Worries were also expressed about those living in poor material circumstances. Mixed views were expressed about the presence of professional carers within the home. Although they were seen to provide much needed support for the informal carer, the presence of 'strangers' was regarded by some as intrusive and compromising of the ideal of 'home'. (460)

While there is an assumption, then, that health and social services are responsible for caring for frail older people at home or in care homes, in this paper I want to question that presumption. This is partly because I bring together the notion that home is connected to dwelling, embodiment and relationality and is much more than just a place to have an existence. As contemporary critiques of health and social services show, the complex conditions of possibility under which practitioners currently practice means that they have been, as Twigg (2000b) puts it, dominated by practical concerns and provision and delivery issues. That is, the home, as a space of care, is all too easily constituted in terms of mere existence.

The critical issue is for more and more people to turn their attention to examining what makes up a life—rather than mere existence—for older people in homes and at home. So it is this issue of quality of life and 'the ideal of home', of what it is like to live in either one's own home or indeed in a residential or nursing home where one is constituted as a 'recipient', or customer, of a substantial amount of nursing and personal care that I want to think through. Specifically, I want to extend Haraway's (1997) thinking over how each being brings a world with them to the question of how we can begin to rethink these situations in terms of what kinds of worlds are being made through what is kept and what is disposed of and how the kinds of worlds that people make together in such situations reproduce or resist the kinds of political, historical and social stabilities discussed above.

MAKING HOME CARE CARE

The issue of how to make health care caring in the home is normally thought through in relation to making care more tailored to individual needs and in terms of matters of choice: policies and processes for enhancing the autonomy, dignity and self-determination of the cared for. For example, Percival (2002) notes that the very construction of the space of a home embodies personal and family-oriented priorities:

> domestic spaces have a significant influence on the scope that older people have to retain a sense of self-determination. It is shown that environmental defects, such as poorly configured domestic spaces, have consequences for older people's sense of continuity and choice. The conclusions are that domestic spaces are living spaces that embody personal and family-oriented priorities. It is suggested that older people require adequate, accessible and personalized domestic spaces in order to facilitate three important objectives: routines, responsibilities and reflection. (729)

Here, Percival helps break down what makes up the sense of being at home as opposed to elsewhere. This includes routines, habits, reflection and family. Critically, home is marked by activities (routines, etc.) but also by a complex web of responsibilities. In addition, Percival stresses how home is also marked by possibilities for reflection.

Percival, like many others (see also Rowles and Chaudhury 2005) is privileging the association between being at home, the construction of space and notions of self-determination, a sense of personal continuity and choice. These are the cultural preoccupations that assert the notion that meaning is tied to the figure of the individual, and the relationships they do or do not have. Also it asserts the possibility of feeling at home as a stable condition.

While I do not want to undermine how important a sense of feeling at home is, it is never as simple as that: grounds and spaces shift, and we, and meaning, get shifted with them. Home is a 'complex location', not a fixed space, but one characterized by ambiguity, tensions and ambivalence. It is also a social construction: an idea, discursively constituted. So while home is usually associated with ontological security, it can become easily threatened and threatening. For example, in Euro-American culture, home is increasingly both a commodity, something to be owned, an investment, as well as something that displays identity. Thus, as an investment, thinking about home may intrude worries and fears regarding finances, repairs and improvements. In addition, home can become a place of threat by being located in a neighborhood that is disturbing (Scharf, Phillipson, and Smith 2003), or in the context of abusive relationships (500,000 older people in the UK are thought to suffer abuse at home, O'Keeffe et al. 2007). And, finally, home may be invaded by relative 'strangers' such as health and social care professionals and assistants and their paraphernalia (Twigg 2000a, 2000b).

Home as such is not just somewhere that someone is by themselves, with their things, their family, their routines and ways, including their choices and their decisions. It is also to be understood as a space that is built, formed of processes and relations, including reflection and present absences. Here one can think about how it is that materials, as well as thoughts, make what is not necessarily present in the home, present (see also Hurdley 2007). Critically, what is peculiar here is how home routed through self and identity can become 'elsewhere' (Derrida and Fathy 2000) through this presence of 'others'.

Thus I want to explore an approach that allows for a perspective that focuses on how a sense of *being at home* as dwelling is accomplished, and I want to connect this to everyday care, not just as a matter of conduct (Latimer 2000) but as a matter of dwelling: being-with as well as being-in-the world. Critiques and examinations such as Gott et al.'s (2004) and Percival's (2002), as important as they are in their focus on the meaning of home, seem to me to be trapped in the idea that meaning can be individuated, simply stabilized, and that homecare, to become more caring, needs to be more respectful of individual selves, particularly in terms of what they already have, who they were and choice. Here several things need unpacking which we can understand as dividing practices, dividing practices with distinct political and ontological effects.

DIVIDING CARE AND DWELLING

There are conditions of possibility that make the association between care and dwelling problematic. First, as mentioned above, there is a conflation of care with provision: the ethical and dynamic dimension of care as embodied, processual, intimate and relational (Letiche 2008) is diminished. Second, the elision between getting old and being static institutes an idea that as you get very old, and increasingly frail, and in need of more and more help, there is a sense in which you are no longer constituted as going anywhere, but as immobile, frozen in the past, without a future (Latimer 1997). Vitality is easily effaced.

In a sense, then, the very old are no longer constituted as persons engaged in what Heidegger (1978) thinks of as "building" or world-forming (Latimer 2009a). It is as if they actually are in a state of withdrawal, rather than that this sense of withdrawal is a socially constructed obligation. And building, as will be seen in this paper, is a part of dwelling, of doing more than existing, eking out a life. This is not just, with contemporary discourse, to emphasize active ageing as the key to life-long wellbeing. Building, as will be seen, is not just a matter of construction, it is a matter of what it is that gets cared for or 'kept'. And building is nothing without thinking, in the sense of thinking with.

Third, there is an absence of recognition that services and interventions can be rethought as a *part of a life*, that is, as building or world-forming, for each person involved. Here I do not just mean the so-called recipients of care, but of each person involved in those activities designated as interventions. Interaction here may include technologies, rituals and events such as are involved in bathing, dressing, washing, walking, medical prescription, assistive technologies and so on and so forth. The difficulty is that there is a division between these things: a separation and specialization of things that nurses do or carers do, and of the carers' involvement in the activity of caring. That is, "the conduct of care" (Latimer 2000, 2003, 2007)—including all the materials in use and how and when they are used, and when they are not, the ways in which people and bodies interact or don't, all that goes to make care up—is as much a part of people making a life, a world together (or not). And, critically, the *how* of conduct is constitutive of the kind of worlds that are being made.

The shift to linking care and the art of dwelling (see also Becker 2008; Bendien 2010; Schillmeier and Domenech 2009) is to help focus how the conduct of care is not something outside of life, provided in order for people to exist and have a life, but something that involves people and things in interaction in ways that are constitutive of a life. That is, care is about building because it is world-forming. Care as being-with and as world-forming may only be a part of what goes to make up a world: the activities are intermittent, people shift extensions and relations, and as they do so, they shift worlds so that their life together at one moment (bathing, walking, getting dressed) only ever "partially connects" (Strathern 1991). After all, even when people occupy the same house and live together over time, their co-presence is intermittent, they go in and out of being together.

KEEPING AND DWELLING: RELATIONAL EXTENSION AND THE IDEA OF HOME

So I am thinking about home and care as a space made up of interactions between persons, materials and technologies. That is, as with all spaces, they are made up of people and things, technologies, discourses and so on and so forth, but that as these come and go, are made present one moment and absent the next, worlds of particular kinds are made and unmade. Here 'things' help make and shift the world as much as people (see also Nelson 2006).

Within this perspective of drawing on Heidegger's notion of dwelling, for living to be more than simply existing requires care:

> . . . the manner in which we humans are on the earth, is *Buan*, dwelling . . . This word *bauen*, however, also means at the same time to cherish, to protect, to preserve and to care for, to till the soil and cultivate the vine. Such building only takes care . . . Building as dwelling, that is, as being on the earth, however, remains for man's everyday experience that which is from the outset "habitual"—we inhabit it . . . (Heidegger 1978, 349)

Heidegger brings to the fore notions of 'keeping', particularly his idea of giving *room* to things. In going on to highlight that this also entails making 'room' for relations, I am seeking to draw *Mitsein* (Being-with) alongside *Dasein* (Being-in-the-world). For Heidegger, an emphasis on *Mitsein* avoids the reduction of relations to those dyadic forms founded upon the division between self and Other.

The point here is to recognize that dwelling is not only grounded within locations: a room, a house, a care home, a neighborhood. Dwelling also takes place as and whenever *relations* are formed in the here and now. As Strathern (1991) shows in her emphasis on extension, relations alter from moment to moment as one set of prosthetic materials is exchanged for another: a telecare alarm, a commode, a wheelchair, a zimmer frame, photos of friends and family, medications, dressings, and so on. These materials can just be *exchanged* in home care contexts as if they are purely functional or personal, provided to support existence or preserved as expressions of self. Or in contrast, these materials can be thought of as forming the extensions with which people have relations with each other. It is attention to things in this latter sense that I want to press in the making up of spaces of care.

This process, what I am calling after Strathern, relational extension (Latimer 2001, 2009a; Munro 1996; Strathern 1991), involves not only the consumption and disposal of 'things' as might be presumed. Nor does it just suppose that attachment to things simply carries self-identity, helping to express who or what a person is or to what they belong (Douglas and Isherwood 1989). For example, how things such as photo albums, a favorite chair or ornament can display choice and identity or can carry a sense of self as 'memories', to help, for example, maintain a sense of personal continuity (Fairhurst 1997), although these are important aspects of attachment to things (Hurdley 2007). Rather, I want to stress how the meaning of things is not just fixed, so that any alteration to extensions is an alteration to relations and performs a shift in *world*. For example, photographs displayed in frames in a room do not just display identity and relations but are a means through which people, as they pick up, look at and/or talk about each others' photos, are making relations with each other. What are simultaneously moved around, passed from one to the other, along with the materials of extension being switched or reordered, are 'attachments' in that other, larger sense. There is thus an 'us-ness' as well as a 'there-ness' to a sense of dwelling; feelings of longing and belonging are affected by the relations created and sustained by giving (or not giving) room to things, and those others that things make present.

All this has implications for the meaning of home, as well as for understandings of self and identity. Here there are two inter-related themes. First, the way in which *the idea of home* can be understood as becoming individuated, ostensibly forming part of one's possessions, or 'capital'. Second, that this meaning of home for Euro-Americans can be seen as gravitating from feelings of belonging being anchored within specific locations to matters of identity becoming entangled in locutions that address notions of self. What is usually thought of as engendering a quality life in the context of home and care is caught in this latter emphasis. So that the way in which 'home' is created and made is something to be determined by the individual, to not only reflect differences in cultural means, but also to suggest a more general shift in trajectory around 'face' rather than 'place'. How older people are provided with care and support is directed by an idea of preserving or conserving face, in terms of self, autonomy and choice, rather than recognizing how all that goes to make up the space of care is implicated in the building of a life, a world, a here and now, a place to dwell. The British poet Philip Larkin catches the displacement of home from locale to self, from place to face, in one of his most acclaimed works, *Mr Bleaney*.[5]

'ROOM' FOR RELATIONS

In its deft imagery Philip Larkin's (1964) poem *Mr Bleaney* locates his characters in the austerity of England in the 1950s, an era in which the British were slowly emerging from post-war rationing. This was a time in which many people felt economically deprived and labor had to keep mobile in order to find work in car factories like "the Bodies," set somewhere in the Midlands. The domestic needs of these transitory men were often met by women householders, sometimes widowed by the recent world war, whose lack of income led them to turn their homes into boarding houses.

His former landlady introduces one of these solitary male lodgers, Mr. Bleaney, in the first stanza of the poem. In the next two stanzas the narrator of the poem locates the surroundings in greater detail, the drabness of the lodgings instantly familiar to any reader in England who had to move away from home and stay in 'digs' for a first job or as a university student. For others the barrenness of the room is recognizable from holidays at the English seaside in Victorian and Edwardian houses offering Bed & Breakfast. Without our ever hearing Mr. Bleaney's version of events, the next two stanzas go on to detail the annual and daily habits of Mr. Bleaney, the narrator's predecessor. Finally, the last two stanzas form the 'movement' of the poem, wherein the narrator, reflecting on finding himself situated within the same set of attachments, imagines a moment in which Mr. Bleaney might also have examined his life.

In taking "Mr Bleaney's room," as the landlady styles the place she is about to let, the narrator is also inheriting something of Mr. Bleaney's life. In the dim light of the naked 60-watt bulb, for instance, he lies on the same "fusty" bed and uses the same "saucer-souvenir" as an ashtray. With only an upright chair to sit on and no "room" for his books or bags, there is little else for the narrator to do but stand looking out at clouds tousled by the wind, or stare at the "thin and frayed" curtains falling five inches short of the windowsill.

This ghostly life is amplified daily by listening to the landlady endlessly recounting the mundane details of Mr. Bleaney's hourly and yearly routine. Almost immediately the narrator picks up on the landlady's expectations that *his* habits should echo those of his predecessor. After all if Mr. Bleaney saw fit to dig over her garden, watch her television downstairs and prefer sauce to gravy, why wouldn't he?

The narrator does not give his reasons for deciding to stay. Nor does he say for how long he expects to lodge in what he calls this "hired box." What we do know, though, is that it cannot be for long. And this is not simply because there are no creature comforts or "room" for books, the tools of his trade. It is the all-enveloping shroud of Mr. Bleaney's life that warns him of the dangers of remaining. For as much as he is being forced to identify with and imagine the life of the person who stayed before him, it is inconceivable to the narrator that anyone could call this "home."

As this paper is about to argue, the issue of locale is never simply one of place rather than space. While conceding residential buildings do indeed provide lodgings, Heidegger (1978, 348) does so only in order for him to insist on dwelling involving much more than mere inhabitation. As he remarks, houses in themselves do not provide any guarantee that dwelling occurs in them. So what does it mean to dwell? To what do we need to give 'room'?

This seems to be the question the narrator of *Mr Bleaney* is asking. Yet in dwelling, in that more negative sense of the word, in stanzas 2 and 3 on the bareness of the locale, the naked 60-watt bulb, the all-too-short and threadbare curtains, and the tussocky, littered building strip for a view, the narrator seems to all but miss just what Bleaney himself has been busy giving 'room' to. Indeed, from a perspective of enhancement—the idea that as we go through life we should make, get, spend [6] —the art of Mr. Bleaney's dwelling is made invisible: it seems the narrator feels that nothing in this locale is *worth* keeping.

What then has Mr. Bleaney been giving 'room' to? Exactly what is it that Mr. Bleaney is keeping? The motivating question of the poem, surely, is not the motif raised in the first two lines of the last stanza, the Thatcherite issue that in renting rather than buying their own box both Bleaney and the narrator are failing to do their bit. It is more to appreciate instead that the poet, if not his narrator, has been asking just what is it that Mr. Bleaney 'admits' into his life? What is it he 'installs' in terms of relations?

In returning to the poem at hand, further reading suggests the narrator has been dismissing almost all Mr. Bleaney does as mere *habit*, a life reduced to the mechanics of routine and repetition:

> I know his habits—what time he came down,
> His preferences for sauce to gravy, why
>
> He kept plugging at the four aways—

Seen from another angle, however, what is clear is that what Mr. Bleaney is good at keeping are *relations*. What he nurtures and sustains, and so safeguards, are the relationships that he has either inherited or established through his routines and habits. This is true of his "yearly frame" in spending Christmas with his sister in Stoke and always returning to the Frinton people to take his summer holidays at the seaside.

It is especially at his lodgings, though, that Mr. Bleaney expands relations. He installs these by keeping up his routines of digging the landlady's garden and by watching television downstairs with her. Despite the narrator's voice, we come to understand how Mr. Bleaney has made himself "at home": not only eating the landlady's meals, but perhaps by sharing many of his thoughts with her. Even, perhaps, to the point of his making out that he prefers the modern conveniences of bottled sauce (HP Brown, Heinz Tomato Ketchup) to her cooking the gravy she might otherwise have felt was necessary to accompany his meals.

The landlady has also made 'room' for Mr. Bleaney beyond his room: she has bought the television "he egged her on to buy" (a real luxury in

1955) and which she appears to continue to keep at the same high volume as when she and he watched together. Apparently she also shared in the knowledge of all those things that gave his life rhythm and meaning: why he bet on the football pools (the "four-aways") and with whom he stayed on his holidays. So much so that Mr. Bleaney, someone who has to be mobile for work and is too poor to own much for himself, has enlarged his ambit beyond his "hired box." And in living rather than lodging, his life so intermingles with his landlady's that it outlasts his stay.

BUILDING 'WORLDS'

In reducing the nature of all Mr. Bleaney's 'extensions' (Latimer 2001; Munro 1996; Strathern 1991) to 'habits', the narrator of the poem appears to have made a fundamental mistake. These are no mere habits: on the contrary, Mr. Bleaney has been an *inhabitant*. He has made his lodgings his dwelling. And in his making 'room' for many things—the garden, the sauce, the telly—relations are enlarged and made more possible. Each activity entails an intermingling through the ways in which he has made his landlady's 'attachments' partially, if temporarily, his own. The care of the garden, the building of a life, is not in his having made anything lasting, or even, as already discussed, in his owning anything; it is the *keeping* up of his routines that matters since it is these that bring about a regular, mundane affirmation of what it is that he cares for.

Where Mr. Bleaney and his landlady made a *world* together, the narrator is more isolated. He finds himself in a 'locale' full of things to which he cannot relate. There is almost nothing, apart from an ashtray and a bed, to which the narrator can attach himself. The telly, the sauce and the garden are almost meaningless to him. In his rejection of these other things *as* Other, the narrator finds he can only lodge; the boarding house can never be his home. For he cannot dwell there: it seems he has no 'room' for the extensions, or relations, that it offers.

It is reasonable to assume in all this that the narrator is using Mr. Bleaney to reflect on the quality of his own life. In this the poem comes to its enigma, its *movement,* in the narrator asking whether or not Mr. Bleaney, when he too was alone in this room, came to realize that:

> . . . how we live measures our own nature,
> And at his age having no more to show
> Than one hired box should make him pretty sure
> He warranted no better . . .

The narrator ends this long, chilling reflection with a crucial caveat: "I don't know."

What the poem communicates in this last stanza is a moment in which the narrator is measuring his own worth. It is no longer Mr. Bleaney's life that is his concern, but his own. For as much as he has stepped, so to speak, into the shoes of his predecessor, he cannot 'follow' him as a figure who has, anthropologically speaking, 'gone before'. And since he cannot so fathom him in this way, he cannot also be sure whether Bleaney ever saw life as bleakly as he, the narrator, is doing in the here and now. Or even be sure Mr. Bleaney has ever stopped to think?

Up to this point the narrator has conducted his reflection in the mode of comparison (cf. Strathern 1997). In this final thought, however, the poem goes beyond the narrator's crisis of worth to realize that, for all he shares some of the selfsame objects of his predecessor's life, the narrator does not know if Mr. Bleaney ever saw himself as the narrator is seeing himself now. He does not know if Mr. Bleaney ever "stood and watched" the "frigid wind," or shivered as he "lay on the fusty bed/ Telling himself that this was home." He does not know whether Mr. Bleaney stopped long enough to reflect on *his* life "without shaking off the dread/ That how we live measures our own nature."

Thus the poem, when first grasped, offers insight into a moment of doubt for the narrator over *his* inability to dwell. His own lack of 'installations' seems to have left him, if wittingly, bereft of any feeling of home. Hence the dramatic shift in the final three words of the poem. The fatal caveat "I don't know" makes a closing that, in turn, creates way for an opening: a re-reading of all the reader has read before.

This is the moment where the poet switches the narrator from making a complacent dismissal of Mr. Bleaney as a man of mere mechanical habits. Instead, lacking a 'home' in the here and now, he seems to realize how Mr. Bleaney's room also portends his own worth—as if there could ever be such a thing as having "our own nature"? In the frisson of self-evaluation, the narrator finds that all that stands between him and "bare life" (cf. Thrift 2004) is his capacity for reflection.

As has been illustrated, the narrator's dwelling is far from being devoid of 'attachment'. Yes, the *route* along which he travels depends upon his refusal of place *as* locale. But what 'takes place' in its place is rather a circular movement of self, an endless shifting of what Goffman (1959) calls front—from 'face' to 'face' to 'face'. And, indeed, such *routes* can be so long installed, so inhabited, that the only 'locale' to which someone like Larkin's narrator can comfortably retreat is towards their own habit of self-reflection.

It seems that 'self' has, not just for Larkin's narrator, become *the* place to dwell, turning the 'world' into a matter of choice, from one moment to the next. This fetishization of self not only helps install the democratics of choice, but incites a constant varying of 'attachments' from one moment to the next—no doubt in order to preserve the illusion of choice. So that what the poem reveals is that there are different 'arts of dwelling' in play. What we 'keep', wittingly or unwittingly, decides our lives.[7] Let me now turn back to the problem of care as provision, and the issue of what is being kept in this constituting of care and of persons.

TELECARE: KEEPING FACE IN PLACE

Telecare is an assistive technology to enable people at risk to stay in their own homes. López and Domenech (2009), in a paper on telecare, describe older peoples' practices around the technologies instituted as part of this health service provision. These technologies manifest a program for conduct that attempts to install ideas in their homes about who they are, as bodies at risk. But for the technology to work the older people have to attach themselves to it: they have to, in my terminology here, 'keep' the paraphernalia that makes up the technology, particularly the emergency call pendant that should be worn 24 hours a day. This requires the older people concerned to behave "as if something dangerous could happen at any time; always wearing the service pendant throughout the house (since you never know when an accident will happen); pressing the green button every 24 hours to advise that all is well; calling once in a while to check that all the information is correct and the devices are working well; installing supplementary devices such as fall detectors in case a sudden fall occurs or medicine dispensers in case at some moment the users do not remember the pills that they have to take." But of course that is not how people live with telecare technology. On the contrary, the older people do not always make room for the things that make the technology up, they can *refuse* them:

> *Interviewer 1:* And, why don't you wear the pendant?
> *Mrs. Carmen:* I don't know, I don't know. I don't know what's wrong, but I don't like it. Now, I've hung it . . . I have a crucifix on the wall behind my bed and I have the pendant there. I do like this (stretches her arm) and I touch it. (laughs)
> *Interviewer 2:* That is to say, you don't like it because you don't like to wear it?
> *Interviewer 1:* Because of aesthetics? Or because . . .
> *Interviewer 2:* Because of aesthetics . . .
> *Interviewer 1:* Does it bother you?
> *Mrs. Carmen:* Not because of aesthetics! No. Because I know that it is something that has to do with . . . I don't know . . . with illness. Or whatever. Doesn't it? I don't like to wear it. (She laughs)
> *Interviewer 2:* Right.
> *Interviewer 1:* That is to say, while you feel fine you prefer to go to the central-telephone and press . . .
> *Mrs. Carmen:* Yes, yes, that's right. Yes.
> *Interviewer 1:* Or would you prefer making the pendant more . . . aesthetic? More . . . like a piece of jewelry?

Mrs. Carmen: It would be the same. The impression would be the same.

Interviewer 1: Right.

Interviewer 2: Right.

Mrs. Carmen: No, no. There are times that I really wear it, because . . . Do you know when I wear it? When?

Interviewer 2: When?

Mrs. Carmen: I'm climbing the stepladder.

Interviewer 2: Right.

Mrs. Carmen: That's when I wear it.

Interviewer 1: When you see that there is danger?

Mrs. Carmen: Yes.

Interviewer 2: That is, when you see that there is a possibility of falling down or . . .

Mrs. Carmen: If I might fall down, I wear it.

Interviewer 2: But when you feel safe, then . . .

Mrs. Carmen: Walking I'm safe. I can fall down, but I don't (she laughs).[8]

(López and Domenech, 187)

So Mrs. Carmen, in Domenech and Lopez's analysis, insists on her interpretations and her autonomy in not completely giving room to the pendant because it represents something to her which does not just change how she lives, but her sense of who she is: it rearranges her face, from someone who is healthy to someone who is ill. In this sense, then, the technology designed to turn the older people around gets turned back by Mrs. Carmen's refusal to keep it as programmed. But what is interesting is that Mrs. Carmen does not see the pendant as in any way performing the relations she has with others: the pendant has no us-ness to it, it seems to exist in a world made up only of Mrs. Carmen as someone who is being constituted as at risk, as someone whose body is failing, but also as someone who is not yet ready to think of herself as ill. So she refuses to let herself become attached to the pendant, to let the pendant rearrange her feelings of self-worth, rather she asserts herself by only becoming partially connected. Here we are in a world of effect and an art of dwelling that routes through face and place.

For a moment, then, like the narrator of *Mr Bleaney*, what gets unconcealed by the technology, even as Mrs. Carmen partially refuses it, is how she is being thrown back on herself and an estimation of her own worth, so that the idea of home routed through face and self gets intensified as something you have to, with remote support, *do on your own*.

SPACES OF CARE AND THE ART OF DWELLING: *THE DIVING BELL AND THE BUTTERFLY*

In this paper I am troubling an approach to homecare as mere provision in order to sustain an existence, however individuated. In my analysis of

Mr Bleaney, I am stressing that there is a need to return to the centrality of being-with in relation to care. Here I have attempted to illuminate how what is kept, and what refused, also performs a shift in 'world' by altering the *relations* we keep. As such it is never only 'things', the prosthetics of extension, that are switched. What are simultaneously moved around are 'attachments' in that other sense; feelings of longing and belonging are affected by the relations that are created and sustained by our giving or not giving 'room' to things like the pendant.

The following analysis is drawn from the film *The Diving Bell and the Butterfly* (Schnabel 2007), a film based on the memoir by Jean-Dominique Bauby (1997). While the subject of the film, Jean-Dominique Bauby (Jean-Do, played by Mathieu Amalric), is a man who is a) young and b) relatively famous, I want to explore what this film helps illustrate about being-with, care and the art of dwelling in the context of home and care for frail older people.

Our protagonist, like many very old and frail people, seems to be locked in—like a deep-sea diver at the bottom of the murky ocean in his metal diving suit. At the age of 43 he has had a massive stroke, has facial palsy, is paralyzed except for being able to blink one eye and breathe through a tracheostomy tube. He seems to be without expectation or hope. He can see, think, hear and remember, but he cannot talk or tell anyone what he wants, nor can he interact with them in any of the usual ways. In the movie we often live in his perspective, looking out at the world as he does, including visualizing and replaying his memories with him.

Through his imagination, his memories and his reactions we learn that he was the antithesis of everything he is now: rich, cool, a playboy, at the heart of the Parisian fashion world (he is the French founding editor of *Elle* magazine), with its emphasis on looks and aesthetics: a prototype of *le beau monde*. He and his life, as it emerges through his reflection, is the apotheosis of liquid life politics (Bauman 2003): lifestyle, consumption, choice, mobility, money, style and the disposability of relationships. He has a lot of face. How he seems now is its opposite: he is stranded, in the arms and at the mercy of others, ugly and incapacitated, imprisoned in the routines and repetitions dictated by his needs. His face has literally and metaphorically collapsed. He is left to reflect as other to his self.

The film shows him with family and with staff in a painstaking effort to build a life in the wreck. But this life becomes, for all involved, much more than the provision of mere existence. There are terrifying moments, such as when, with him, the audience experiences the eyelids of the eye that can no longer blink being sutured together by an insensitive surgeon as he jovially recounts his marvelous skiing holiday: summoning up a glamorous, invigorating world of snow and speed and light that Jean-Do himself enjoyed in the past but which he is now excluded from. There are also extraordinarily humorous moments, such as when Jean-Do is watching his football team about to score the winning goal and a care assistant turns the TV off.

What the film preserves is the shifting of worlds: between a world that is rooted through self, choice and face, and something else, something that stresses relationality. People try to preserve his face by checking what Jean-Do wants, giving him choice and information: blink once for yes and twice for no. "Do you want to see your children?"—two blinks—"No." And so on and so forth, but this cannot completely work; for him to have a life there has to be more. Then there is a moment in the film in which Jean-Do is turned over.

In this moment the speech therapist (Henriette) arrives with her new technology: a card with the letters of the alphabet inscribed on it which she holds up for Jean-Do to see out of his one good eye. She has told Jean-Do that this is for her the most important case she has ever had and that she is determined to make a success of it. Henriette has devised an alphabet in the order that letters most commonly appear. She speaks each letter in its turn in this special order and when she reaches the right letter Jean-Do has to blink. In this way they can build words (and worlds) together. She tells him he must think ahead about what it is that he will want to say in their session.

We see them try out the new technology and become at odds. It is hard for him to concentrate and she goes too fast: it all seems unnatural to him. After some disastrous interactions with his wife and other carers, Jean-Do is in the next session with Henriette when he painfully, letter by letter, blink by blink, spells out the words "I want to die." As he blinks each letter into being it is vocalized by the therapist: i, w, a, n, and so on. All the emotion that Henriette feels as she realizes with horror what he is trying to express cathects[9] (Goffman 1955) her face—and of course we are seeing her face, and its meaning, as Jean-Do sees it, as a portrait of intense emotion and agitation. She then tells him that what he is saying is obscene, that she has only known him a short time but that she already loves him, and that none of it (the situation) is just about him. Hastily she gets up and leaves the room.

We sit with Jean-Do looking at the closed door. She then walks back through it, walks back over to stand in front of him and apologizes, saying she was out of order. The next shot cuts to the two of them huddled together outside working with the alphabet: we are seeing them from our own perspective—not Jean-Do's. From this moment on in the film Jean-Do, his friends, his family, colleagues, are all seen working with the alphabet. I want to suggest that through attaching themselves to the alphabet technology they make relations and build a world together, one in which Jean-Do himself is a vital participant.

At first Jean-Do will not attach himself to the speech therapist's technology. In refusing the extension that the technology offers, he seems at first to be making a choice and asserting his self, and like Mrs. Carmen, refusing the world and the refiguring of his identity that the technology brings with it. At the moment he attaches to the technology and expresses all that he feels, there is a moment in which he, and Henriette, are turned over. In giving room to the technology, they give room to each other—they are both extended through the technology. But in a shocking moment what gets revealed is that he and his care is as much about her life as his. Jean-Do is stunned—it is as if he has never been in a world like this before. Henriette is also deeply shocked. Both he and Henriette are not just turned around, they are turned over (Munro and Belova 2009). What is unconcealed is not just a world of provision and recipience, of effects, but of affect and relationality. They of course go on to perfect the technology, and Jean-Do goes on to write his book before he dies, the book upon which the film is based. Even his memories change, in fact he re-members himself differently, not as the playboy of the western world, but in other kinds of situations, such as shaving his old father.

So at the heart of the (re)building is a gift, the development of a special technology, one that begins to become, at moments, everyone's extension through which they have relations with one another: staff, family friends, publisher, ex-wife, Jean-Do, bringing him and them into touch (Letiche 2009, drawing on Merleau-Ponty). Through the relational extension afforded by the technology, the book that the film is based on is written. This technology, in complete contrast to the pendant partially refused by Mrs. Carmen in Lopez and Domenech's study, is able to reorder the world because of how Jean-Do and his speech therapist and others attach to it and through it. The technology is thus functional, effective and affective. But, critically, as people attach themselves to the technology, they are giving it room and are keeping something that opens them and the space up to dwelling as world-forming: what gets unconcealed is how the space of care is as much a life for practitioners and family as it is for Jean-Do himself. What is usually denied, hidden in health care contexts, is for a moment revealed. And it this possibility of being-with and world-forming that I see in this moment in the film—the moment of the movement in the film from face to locale, from existing to the possibility of dwelling, and one that brings reflection alongside building.

AKROPOLIS AND THE 5 CATS

Some theorists suggest that nursing and caring are about organizing, providing and delivering interventions (e.g., Nelson 2006). And there is no doubt care located as ethical expertise in individuals is deeply problematic. But care does not have to be so limited. What I am stressing here is not just that the affective has been made invisible to analyses of home care or even that "sentimental work" (Strauss et al. 1982) has been simply backgrounded in the pursuit of demonstrable gains. Rather, it is to emphasize being-with and world forming and the possibility that work, care and life are indivisible for both the frail and practitioners alike.

Drawing on a number of sources, including film and literature, as well as ethnographic description, I have explored ideas of home and care in relation to theories of relational extension, including body-world relations, and Heidegger's writing on the art of dwelling. In drawing on an exegesis of a famous poem by Philip Larkin, *Mr Bleaney*, I have illustrated how routines and habits and what we keep are important, but how their importance does not just come from their being personal or functional, but as critical to the making up of home as *Mitsein* or being-with. I then illustrated the mysterious space of care and its possibility for dwelling, and the making and unmaking of worlds together, through a brief excerpt from the film the *Diving Bell and the Butterfly*. I then analyzed this excerpt for how it helps illustrate care and the art of dwelling.

I have wanted to bring into view methods, narratives and discourses that circulate people and difference in ways that help deconstruct the old hierarchies and worries about care, to circulate ways to value both the aged and the frail as people who can be engaged in world-forming. Here, drawing together Strathern's stress on relationality with Martin Heidegger's theory of dwelling, I am not just stressing embodiment but relational extension and would like to press for forms of organization embedded in a view of care routed in body-world relations. Within this view I am pressing that there can be vitality in frailty and that helplessness is not just a condition that inheres in the frail. Helplessness is, as Deddie helps us to understand, relational: it is a construction of the interaction of a person and his or her environment, a body-world relation. My example from the film about Jean-Do helps illustrate this point: that there can be vitality in frailty.

Critically then, there is a need to press for forms of organization that recognize and make available alternative discourses to those which route quality only through face, place and self. Here what is kept (a pendant, a speech therapy technology) can be understood as having the possibility for engaging the frail *and* practitioners in *Mitsein*, in the art of dwelling as world-forming a space of care.

Rather than thinking care simply as provision in the fulfillment of needs, however individuated, even where this is directed at maintaining face, self and choice, a space of care can be rethought for how it affords people (staff, patients, family, friends) a life of creativity, vitality and building, no matter how frail some participants are. The point is how to organize spaces of home care in terms of bringing being-with (*Mitsein*) alongside being-in-the-world, to think home care in ways that switch between privileging the idea of locale and relationality and the emphasis on individuality, face and self. It is possible, but it requires different imaginaries to those put into play through care-as-provision.

Recently I have been engaged in research with colleagues in Humanitas in the Netherlands and have visited one of their communities for elderly people, Akropolis. I want to end with a story from Akropolis to illustrate an approach that helps us to see that what is kept decides our lives, but that keeping is as much to do with *Mitsein*, affect and building as with effects, and face, self, and choice. Akropolis consists of several different spaces: it is like a communal undercover 'open' village, with hairdressers, an internet café, a restaurant, a bar, places to sit and talk and large artifacts, or conversation pieces, such as huge Buddhas or totem poles, a memory museum (Bendien 2010) and individual apartments for couples or singles. It is a charity funded by public and private finance initiatives, and the residents are from less well-off backgrounds. People, as their need for care intensifies, simply receive more care; they do not have to move to another facility. The philosophy of Akropolis is to emphasize the art of living and not health and safety needs. The key strategic principles are happiness, community, privacy and family, with carers and residents constituted as family. Carers are not permitted to just say no to a resident's wishes: like Jean-Do and the speech therapist, they have to find a way together.

An elderly woman wanted to come and live at Akropolis, and she wanted to bring her five cats. In this case after much discussion and dialogue, and organizing, it was agreed that one cat who was very old (aged 21)and frail himself should (ironically) be put down, two cats should go to live with another resident who would love to have the cats and who lived two apartments along from the new resident's allocated apartment, so the cats would be near enough for the new resident to meet with her cats every day; the other two cats would go on living with the new resident in her new apartment. My point is that the disposal as well as the keeping of (and being with) the cats, in many small ways, could not but help reorder the world of Akropolis.

NOTES

1. This is the objective of many of the authors in a recent book (Latimer and Schillmeier 2009), including new perspectives on spaces of care, the frail, especially those with dementia and other (dis)abilities, as well as those who are 'locked in' (e.g., Kraeftner and Kröell 2009, Letiche 2009, Schillmeier 2009).

2. "There is no clear consensus on the definition of frailty; however, it is proposed that frailty comprises a collection of biomedical factors which influences an individual's physiological state in a way that reduces his or her capacity to withstand environmental stresses. Only a subset of older people are at risk of becoming frail; thse are vulnerable, prone to dependency and have reduced life expectancy" (Lally and Crome 2007, 16).

3. We acknowledge the kind permission of Rolland Munro to reproduce this analysis here.

4. Just like other businesses, nursing and residential homes, as well as private home care and telecare providers, can fail or be sold, so that the residents may find that rather than moving to somewhere or being provided with care in ways that they can feel themselves at home 'for life' in they may very well have to be moved on. In addition, older people, as their mobility and capacity for self-care decreases, may become inappropriate for residential or home

care and may need to be moved into a nursing home in which they can receive more and more support.

5. The poem can be read and listened to at http://www.poetryarchive.org/poet-ryarchive/singlePoem.do?poemId=7077 (accessed January 25, 2011).
6. Reflecting William Wordsworth's (1999) famous lines:
    The world is too much with us; late and soon,
    Getting and spending, we lay waste our powers.
7. That the trope of keeping does not exhaust the possibilities here is brought out in Schillmeier's (2009) reading of Heidegger (1978) in terms of what 'stays'. We find this to be a fruitful way of also rethinking dwelling which further research might pursue.
8. Excerpt of an interview with Mrs. Carmen, a user of a telecare service. Mrs. Carmen, 75 y.o., is living alone in the center of Barcelona. She has no contact with her family and her only aid is the visit of a caregiver twice a week.
9. Project emotional energy.

REFERENCES

Audit Commission. 2004. *Support for carers of older people. Independence and well-being.* http://www.audit-commission.gov.uk/reports/NATION-AL-REPORT.asp?CategoryID=&ProdID=93DF6B31-4A50-46bb-B08B-69-DE7C292A60

Bauby, Jean-Dominique. 1997. *The diving bell and the butterfly.* New York: Knopf.

Bauman, Zymunt. 2003. *Liquid love.* Cambridge: Polity Press.

BBC Radio 4. 2008. Care home life is 'slow death'. *Today*, June 4. http://news.bbc.co.uk/today/hi/today/newsid_7408000/7408110.stm

Becker H. 2008. *The art of living in old age.* http://translate.google.com/translate?hl=en&sl=nl&u=http://www.humanitas.nu/&ei=qq3TSZvCFdmZjAeVotTkBg&sa=X&oi=translate&resnum=1&ct=result&prev=/search%3Fq%3D www.humanitas.nu%26hl%3Den%26safe%3Doff%26client%3Dsafari%26rls%3Den

Bendien, Elena. 2010. *From the art of remembering to the craft of ageing.* Published PhD thesis. Humanistik University, Utrecht, NL.

Budlender Debbie. 2008. *The statistical evidence on care and non-care work across six nations.* http://www.unrisd.org/unrisd/website/document.nsf/8b18431d756b708580256b6400399775/f9fec4ea774573e7c1257560003a96b2/$FILE/Budlender2008.pdf.

Cohen, Anthony. 1994. *Self-consciousness: An alternative anthropology of identity.* London: Routledge.

Commission for Social Care Inspection. 2008. *The state of social care in England 2007–08.* www.csci.org.uk

Derrida, Jacques, and Safaa Fathy. 2000. *Tourner les mots: Au bord d'un film.* Paris: Galilée.

Disabled Living Foundation. 2008. *Ethical issues with assistive technology.* http://www.livingmadeeasy.org.uk/scenario.php?csid=43

Douglas, Mary, and Baron Isherwood. 1989. *A world of goods.* Harmandsworth, England: Penguin Books.

Doyle, Martha, and Virpi Timonen. 2009. The different faces of care work: understanding the experiences of the multi-cultural care workforce. *Ageing and Society* 29: 337–350 .

Fairhurst, Eileen. 1997. Recalling life: Analytical issues in the use of memories. In *Critical approaches to ageing and later life,* edited by Anne Jamieson, Sarah Harper and Christina Victor, 62–76. Buckingham: Open University Press.

Featherstone, Mike. 1982. The body in consumer culture. *Theory, Culture & Society* 1(2): 18–33.

Goffman, Erving. 1955. On face-work: an analysis of ritual elements in social interaction. *Psychiatry: Journal of Interpersonal Relations* 18(3): 213–231.

——— 1959. *The presentation of self in everyday life.* New York: Doubleday.

——— 1963. *Stigma: Management of a spoiled identity.* London: Penguin.

——— 1966. [1963]. *Behaviour in public places.* New York: The Free Press.

Gott, M., and J. Seymour, G. Bellamy, S. Ahmedzhai and D. Clark. 2004. Older people's views about home as a place of care at the end of life. *Palliative Medicine* 18: 460–467.

Haraway, Donna. 1997. *Modest–Witness@Second–Millennium. FemaleMan–Meets–OncoMouse: Feminism and technoscience.* With illustrations by Lynne Randolph. London: Routledge.

Heidegger, Martin. 1962. *Being and time,* translated by J. Macquarrie and E. Robinson. Oxford: Basil Blackwell.

——— 1978. Building, dwelling, thinking. In *Basic writings,* edited by D. F. Krell. Translated by Albert Hofstadler. London: Routledge.

Help the Aged. 2009. *Older people in the UK.* Http://Www.Helptheaged.Org.Uk/Nr/Rdonlyres/318e26ca-F4eb-4a91-B77c-A2867f85af63/0/Uk_Facts.Pdf.

Hillman, A. 2008. Social exclusion and the contemporary organisation of health care: An ethnography of older people in Accident and Emergency, unpublished PhD thesis, School of Social Sciences, Cardiff University.

Hurdley, Rachel. 2006. Dismantling mantelpieces: Consumption as spectacle and shaper of self in the home, unpublished PhD thesis, School of City and Regional Planning, Cardiff University.

——— 2007. Objecting relations: the problem of the gift. *The Sociological Review* 55(1): 124–143.

Kraeftner, Bernd, and Judith Kröell. 2009 Washing and assessing: Multiple diagnosis and hidden talents. In *Un/knowing bodies,* edited by Joanna Latimer and Michael Schillmeier, 159–180. Sociological Review Monograph. Oxford: Blackwell.

Lally, Frank and Peter Crome. 2007. Understanding frailty. *Postgraduate Medicine* 83: 16–20.

Larkin, Phillip. 1964. *Mr Bleaney.* In *The Whitsun weddings.* London: Faber & Faber.

Latimer, Joanna. 1997. Giving patients a future: the constituting of classes in an acute medical unit. *Sociology of Health and Illness* 19(2): 160–185.

——— 1999. The dark at the bottom of the stair: participation and performance of older people in hospital. *Medical Anthropology Quarterly* 13(2): 186–213.

——— 2000. *The conduct of care: Understanding nursing practice.* Oxford: Blackwell Science.

——— 2001. All-consuming passions: Materials and subjectivity in the age of enhancement. In *The Consumption of Mass,* edited by Nick Lee and Rolland Munro, 158–173. Sociological Review Monograph. Oxford: Blackwell.

——— 2003. Studying the women in white. In *Advanced Qualitative Research for Nursing,* edited by Joanna Latimer, 231–247. Oxford: Blackwell.

——— 2007. Critical constructionism in nursing research. In *Handbook of Constructionist Research,* edited by J. Holstein and Jay Gubrium, 153–170. New York: Guilford Press.

——— 2009a. Introduction: body, knowledge, world. In *Un/knowing bodies,* edited by Joanna Latimer and Michael Schillmeier, 1–22. Sociological Review Monograph. Oxford: Blackwell.

———— 2009b. Unsettling bodies: Frida Kahlo's portraits and *in/dividuality*. In *Un/knowing bodies,* edited by Joanna Latimer and Michael Schillmeier, 46–62. Sociological Review Monograph. Oxford: Blackwell.

———— 2009c. Care in the era of the gene. Plenary Paper. Governing the Self in the Community and the Clinic, 3rd International in Sickness & In Health Conference, Victoria, BC, Canada, April 15–17, 2009.

———— 2010. Growing old and the art of dwelling: Frailty, participation and social inclusion. Keynote. UN International Day of Older Persons celebratory conference, Cardiff University, September 30.

Latimer, Joanna and Rolland Munro. 2006. Driving the social. In *Against automobility,* edited by Stephen Bohm, Campbell Jones, Chris Land and Matthew Patterson, 32–55. Special Issue: Sociological Review Monograph Series, 54 (s1). Oxford: Wiley-Blackwell. http://onlinelibrary.wiley.com/doi/10.1111/sore.2006.54.issue-s1/issueto.

———— 2009. Keeping and dwelling: relational extension and the idea of home. *Space and Culture* 12(3): 317–331.

Latimer, Joanna, and Michael Schillmeier. Editors. 2009. *Un/knowing bodies.* Special Issue: Sociological Review Monograph Series. Oxford: Wiley-Blackwell.

Letiche, Hugo. 2008. *Making healthcare care,* with a contribution by J. Latimer. Charlotte, NC: IAP.

———— 2009. Bodily chiasms. In *Un/knowing bodies,* edited by Joanna Latimer and Michael Schillmeier, 63–83. Sociological Review Monograph. Oxford: Blackwell.

Lopez, Daniel, and Miquel Domenech. 2009. Embodying autonomy in a home telecare service. In *Un/knowing bodies,* edited by Joanna Latimer and Michael Schillmeier, 181–195. Sociological Review Monograph. Oxford: Blackwell.

May, Carl, and Christine Fleming. 1997. The professional imagination: narrative and the symbolic boundaries between medicine and nursing. *Journal of Advanced Nursing* 25(5): 1094–1100.

Miller, D. 2001. *Home possessions: Material culture behind closed doors.* Oxford: Berg.

Munro, Rolland. 1996. A consumption view of self: Extension, exchange and identity. In *Consumption matters: The production and experience of consumption,* edited by Stephen Edgell, Kevin Hetherington and Alan Warde, 248–273. Oxford: Blackwell.

Munro, Rolland, and Olga Belova. 2009 The body in time: Knowing bodies and the "interruption" of narrative. In *Un/knowing bodies,* edited by Joanna Latimer and Michael Schillmeier, 87–99. Sociological Review Monograph. Oxford: Blackwell.

Myerhoff, Barbara. 1978. *Number our days.* New York: Simon and Schuster.

NHS Information Centre. 2006. *Community care statistics 2005: Home help and care services for adults, England.* http://www.ic.nhs.uk/statistics-and-data-collections/social-care/adult-social-care-information/community-care-statistics-2005:-help-and-care-services-for-adults-england.

Nelson, Siobhan. 2006. Ethical expertise and the problem of the good nurse. In *The complexities of care: Nursing reconsidered,* edited by Siobhan Nelson and Suzanne Gordon, 69–87. Ithaca: Cornell University Press.

Office for Fair Trading (OFT). 2005. *Care homes for older people in the UK. A market study.* http://www.oft.gov.uk/shared_oft/reports/consumer_protection/oft780.pdf.

O'Keeffe, M., A. Hills, M. Doyle, C. McCreadie, S. Scholes, R. Constantine, A. Tinker, J. Manthorpe, S. Biggs and B. Erens. 2007. *UK Study of Abuse and*

Neglect of Older People. Research Findings. London: King's College London; National Centre for Social Research.

Papadopoulos, Dimitris, Niamh Stephenson and Vassilis Tsianos. 2008. *Escape routes: Control and subversion in the 21st century*. London: Pluto Press.

Percival, John. 2002. Domestic spaces: Uses and meanings in the daily lives of older people. *Ageing & Society* 22: 729–749.

Relatives and Residents Association, The. 2009. *Charity questions Commission for Social Care Inspection (CSCI)'s report of improvement in care home standards*. http://www.relres.org/pdf/press-releases-articles/R&RA_press_release_270109.pdf

Rowles, Graham, and Habib Chaudhury. Editors. 2005. *Home and identity in late life: International perspectives*. New York: Springer Publishing Company.

Rudge, Trudy. 2009. Beyond caring? Discounting the differently known body. In *Un/knowing bodies*, edited by Joanna Latimer and Michael Schillmeier, 233–248. Sociological Review Monograph. Oxford: Blackwell.

Savage, J. 1995. *Nursing intimacy*. London: Scutari Press.

Scharf, Thomas, Chris Phillipson and Alison Smith. 2003. Older people's perceptions of the neighbourhood: Evidence from socially deprived urban areas. *Sociological Research Online*, 8(4): http://www.socresonline.org.uk/8/4/scharf.html.

Schillmeier, Michael. 2009. Actor-networks of dementia. In *Un/knowing bodies*, edited by Joanna Latimer and Michael Schillmeier, 141–158. Sociological Review Monograph. Oxford: Blackwell.

Schillmeier, Michael and Miquel Domènech. 2009. Care and the art of dwelling: Bodies, technologies, and home. *Space and Culture* 12: 288–291.

Schnabel, Julian. Director. 2007. *The Diving Bell and the Butterfly* (Le scaphandre et le papillon, *original title*). Screenplay by Ronald Harwood; produced by Jon Kilik, Kathleen Kennedy and Pierre Grunstein; executive producers Jim Lemley and Leonard Glowinski. Miramax Films Inc.

Schofield, I. 2008. An exploration of how delirium in older people is explained and understood by qualified nurses. Unpublished PhD thesis. Glasgow Caledonian University.

Skeggs, Beverly. 2004. *Class, self, culture*. London: Routledge.

Strathern, Marilyn. 1988. *The gender of the gift*. Berkeley: University of California Press.

——— 1991. *Partial connections*. Savage, MD: Rowman & Littlefield.

——— 1992. *After nature: English kinship in the late twentieth century*. Cambridge: Cambridge University Press.

——— 1993. *The relation: Issues in complexity and scale*. Cambridge, UK: Prickly Pear Press.

——— 1997. Gender: Division or comparison? In *Ideas of Difference: Social Spaces and the Labour of Division*, edited by Kevin Hetherington and Rolland Munro, 42–63. Sociological Review Monograph. Oxford: Blackwell Publishers.

Strauss, Anselm, S. Fagerhaugh, B. Suszek and C. Wiener. 1982. Sentimental work in the technologised hospital. *Sociology of Health and Illness* 4(3): 254–278.

Thrift, Nigel. 2004. Bare life. In *Cultural bodies: Ethnography and theory*, edited by Helen Thomas and Jamilah Ahmed, 145–169. Oxford: Blackwell.

Tulle, Emmanuelle. 2008. The ageing body and the ontology of ageing: athletic competence in later life. *Body & Society* 14(3): 1–19.

Twigg, Julia. 2000a. Carework as a form of bodywork. *Ageing and Society* 20: 389–411.

——— 2000b. *Bathing—the body and community care*. London: Routledge.

Wiles, Janine. 2005. Home as a new site of care provision and consumption. In *Ageing & place. Perspectives, policy, practice*, edited by Gavin J. Andrews and David R. Phillips, 79–97. London: Routledge.

Wordsworth, William. 1999 [1888]. *The Complete Poetical Works*. London: Macmillan and Co; http://www.bartleby.com/145/ww317.html

3 Homes for Care
Reconfiguring Care Relations and Practices

Isabel Dyck and Kim England

The devolution of long-term health and social care into the homes of Canadians is changing the meanings, physical conditions and spatio-temporal ordering of both domestic life and health care work in such homes. When services are required for months or even years, the home must function simultaneously as a personal dwelling, a setting for domestic life and a site for complex, labor-intensive care work. Blurring the boundary between the public sector of health care and the private sphere of the home may well be cost-saving from the perspective of the state but brings into play a set of dynamics that complicates the transference of professional and institutional functions and discourses into homespace. Furthermore, the returning of care to the home discounts the heterogeneity of homespaces within which care is provided, not only in terms of the home's materiality, but also as a space redolent with social and symbolic meanings.

In this chapter, we take up the heterogeneity of homespace and the various tensions between the 'public' and 'private' in the context of the provision of long-term home care services in Ontario, Canada. These services allow the frail elderly and people living with chronic illnesses or disabilities to stay in their homes and age 'in place'. Mol (2008) and others have recognized the complexity of care relations and practices, and here we expand on such analyses. We draw on interviews and visual data taken from a multi-disciplinary project, which focused on the conditions and dynamics underpinning care in the home. Using a mix of methods, although primarily qualitative, the study explored the different experiences of care giving and receiving, the material conditions of the home and the meaning of home to different sets of participants in the research. We take the home to be a material and discursive site, with its spatial arrangements, location, amenities and furnishings interpreted through discursive constructions of 'family', gender, health/illness, ability/disability that frame dominant representations of the home.

In the analysis we focus on the micro dynamics of care to explore how homespaces are 'brought into being' as caregiving spaces through the practices of routinized care. Informed by Foucault's ideas on disciplinary power, our analysis argues that care spaces are constructed, negotiated and maintained through spatialized social and material practices of power and resistance. These practices are performed within specific discursive fields, social interactions and inanimate objects that signal a particular ethic of care.

The chapter is organized as follows: we begin with a brief discussion of themes within the care literature pertinent to our argument. We provide a short description of the study's methods to indicate the source of our data, following this with a section on general features of working conditions for paid care workers and how these provide ambiguities and tensions for the practices of care giving in the home. This acts as a context for the case study we use to unpack the various dynamics and practices in play as a home is 'brought into being' as a carespace. We conclude with comments is on how the practices and processes discussed may contribute to understanding of the home as a specific spatiality of an ethic of care.

CARESCAPES, POWER AND AN ETHIC OF CARE

The home is now an established component of contemporary carescapes, which bring together various sets of players into the orchestration and practice of long-term health and social care (Barnett 2005). The emergence of the home as a central site in the provision of care necessarily shifts how paid care can be delivered, including how spaces of care may be reconfigured as they function as both a paid workplace and the care recipient's home. While the home may be viewed as a micro-scale materiality, in fact it is also deeply inflected by relations originating in sites and scales beyond its material boundaries. Nettleton and Burrows (1994) for example, describe the location of care in the home as a "re-spatialisation" of disciplinary power as the state manages particular bodies—bodies defined in terms of their frailty or disability or the failing bodies of the chronically and/or terminally ill. Certainly the tentacles of the state, in the form of policy guidelines and directives, reach deep into the organization and daily practices of care and the formation of care relations in the site of the home (England and Dyck 2011a). Care agency constraints on time allocated to tasks and the legal demarcation of job category boundaries, for example, set a context in which care is delineated in scope and content.

Another strand of literature, particularly when informed by feminist scholarship, is the elaboration of care as a relation, specifically in the context of the notion of an ethic of care. Tronto (Fisher and Tronto 1990; Tronto 1993) has been especially influential in putting forward a research agenda concerning how we might think of ethical care. Her concept of care is intended to provide a broad framework for moral, political and policy decisions, but has resonance for our specific focus on home-based care. Here the well-rehearsed distinction between 'caring about' (relational, therapeutic emotional labor) and 'caring for' (task-oriented, physical labor) comes into play. This distinction refers to the analytic separation (although empirically they may overlap) of the emotional dimension of a care relationship and the physical tasks of care work, such as those of 'high touch', intimate body work. Healey (2008) comments on family caregiving as an ethical act; family caregivers do not necessarily see it as an obligation or burden. Here we see the overlap of caring about and caring for. There is little work on formal care providers in similar terms, although Bondi (2008) emphasizes the importance of addressing the relationality of caregiving work—a relationship between paid care worker and care receiver that will be power-inflected and emotionally laden.

In home care work, the paid care worker/care recipient relation differs from that in the institutional setting of a hospital or long-term care facility. The worker's workplace is the care recipient's home and home health care work blurs the boundaries between home and paid work, further complicating the work relation. Meanings of the home are destabilized as it becomes a workplace for the paid caregiver while also remaining central to a care recipient's sense of identity and everyday routines. The work relation has a greater potential to be shaped by intimacy, affective labor, ideologies of the family, as well as public discourses about health care in the home setting. Dyck et al. (2005) explore the negotiation of this relationship, focusing on the material, social and symbolic reconstructions of home. Their focus is primarily on the care recipient. In this chapter we take up the perspective of the paid care workers to help explicate more fully how attention to the practices of care can give insight into the emotional and power-inflected relationships that underwrite the constitution of the home as a carespace. We consider how the intertwining of the materialities of home, employment contracts and the emotional dimension of care complicate the notion of ethical caregiving. In effect, we are dealing with a set of work relations that are complicated by antagonisms and ambiguities based on the merging of 'public' work and 'private' home spheres, including their emotional complexity.

The Study

Data for our analysis are drawn from a broad scope study on home care, which placed the home as central to the organization and experience of care giving and care receiving. It was conducted by a research team including sociologists, nurse researchers and geographers.[1] Sub-teams explored the experiences of paid care workers, family caregivers and care receivers, along with a detailed investigation of the various homespaces of care recipient participants in the project. Seventeen cases were recruited in both urban and rural areas of Ontario. These included some children, but care recipients were primarily adults with chronic illness or disability. This chapter draws only on adult cases. Analysis involved coding of interview transcripts and field notes, with cross-comparison across cases. Initially we will draw on a range of cases to make our general points, but later in the chapter focus particularly on one case to draw out the processual dynamics of constituting carespace. This allows us to trace detail within the case to elaborate the articulation of local and wider processes signaled in the thematic analysis of the interview transcripts.

FRAMING HOME CARE: CONTEXTS, MATERIALITIES AND EMBODIED PRACTICES

Structuring Care

The context of the study—Ontario, Canada—is one where restructuring of home care since the mid-1980s has incorporated managed competition. The province was divided into Community Care Access Centres (called CCACs), which are regionally based organizations that govern the delivery of home care services and assess potential clients needs for care services in their region. Agencies delivering home care services now compete for contracts from the CCAC. The introduction of managed competition into home care ushered in a number of large, private, for-profit corporations that in some parts of the province came to control the majority of the market-share at the expense of non-profit organizations, such as the Victorian Order of Nurses that had provided home nursing services for decades. Managed competition is not only put into practice at the level of policy-making but it also impacts upon the work experiences of those whose job it is to provide care to the care recipient, sometimes on a daily basis. Paid care work can be rewarding, but the introduction of managed competition means more and different work for workers, increasing workloads and increasing stress. Cost-savings have been achieved by reducing the number of visits by home care workers and reducing the duration of those visits. This has also been the case for non-profit agencies that increased the workloads of their workers, which for many meant more stress and less job satisfaction (Armstrong and Armstrong 2003; Aronson and Neysmith 1997; England et al. 2007).

Working Conditions, Practicing Care

In addition to the effects of community care organization on the day-to-day demands made on paid care workers, the specific materialities of homes may sometimes present difficult conditions or raise ambiguities for care workers as they perform their work. Furthermore, the emotional dimensions of care work are sharpened in the home setting. Finally, agency regulations also shape what happens in the home as workplace, setting limits, for example, on time allocated to specific tasks or a limit on what tasks are covered in a care package. Such regulations may place workers in a dilemma if they perceive a resultant compromise in the quality of care provided. These three aspects of care provision in the home are signaled below.

Given the high correlation between disabling health conditions and poverty, high demands are exacted from households in which living, working and housing conditions may be less than optimal because space and amenities are scarce and resources are stretched or absent (McKeever et al. 2006). Homes are not designed as healthcare spaces, and while some provide adequate working conditions for care workers (and family caregivers), others do not.

Some homes in the study were cluttered and cramped, with doorways too narrow for wheelchairs or for client-lifting equipment, and may have limited space for workers to prepare medications or bathe clients. However, there were also homes that had been renovated to accommodate the client's care needs (for example, ramps, roll-in showers and an intercom system), or the family was affluent enough to move to more appropriate housing.

For workers, care recipients and family members, homespace becomes a space of ambiguity, with tensions between its designation as a site for paid care and as a home where private lives are conducted outside the view of the public eye. The following examples show how such ambiguity is expressed by care workers and clients, and how professional performance signifiers may be compromised. For example, a physiotherapist indicates the way social norms associated with entering a home as private space can complicate a worker's positioning:

> I take off my shoes. Ahm, but it's something you're not quite comfortable with, I'm a professional. I'm professionally dressed, I'm treating them, giving them medical advice, and standing in my socks . . . I find that a little weird.

Another worker, a Registered Practical Nurse (RPN), comments on the poor working conditions of one home:

> I have never been in such a filthy home in my entire life . . . it bothered me from the first day I went in and it bothers me every time I go in. It's unbelievably dirty . . . And I've always felt unsafe that way because of the uncleanliness.

At the same time, care recipients note the uneasy mix of public and private life, which is reflected in the organization and care of home space:

> It's very, very difficult to open your door to somebody and then in your own home, you know, have a shower or a bowel treatment with a total stranger.

In one home a notice over the wash basin directed at care workers coming into the home signals this reduction in privacy: "Please make sure that the taps are completely off."

Other issues emerge due to the specific location of some homes in rural areas where the quality of the water supply is unpredictable, especially in the summer. Home care regulations are generally not sensitive to the particularities of locality and can create additional tensions for workers, exemplified in the following quotes:

> [T]hey have a [policy] for dressings right now where they won't supply sterile bottles of saline, you know. Well, if you tried to make sterile saline with [client's] water, it comes out rusty brown, and, ah, you know, it's terrible. You wouldn't want to be putting that in a wound. (nurse employed in a rural area)

> She needed care and she didn't have any water, so we used to haul the water from the Laundromat . . . And then the office says we're not allowed to do that . . . but what are you supposed to do? (nurse employed in a rural area)

Such quotes indicate an unsettling of established meanings of 'home' and 'work' which need to be negotiated through the everyday practices of care work.

Despite difficult work conditions in some homes and, in some instances, a client's dissatisfaction with work done, many of the nurses and homemakers drew on discourses of family and friendship in describing a relationship with clients. Such comment indicated a positive affective climate for the provision of care. For example:

> Like you're part of the—you become part of the family . . . I just think that we're friends after all this, all this time. Like she wants to know what's going on with my kids all the time. . . . They're very much part of her existence. (nurse)

One worker, a homemaker without health care training, saw the content of her work as consistent with 'mothering work', seeing her own experience of reproductive work in her own home as transferable to working for clients in their homes. She commented:

> I can say that I am . . . a very skillful homemaker. . . . I haven't taken a course, so I . . . the only thing that I did, I apply everything that I know already to do at home, into . . . her home. (homemaker)

These comments suggest that care provision in the home includes a dimension different from that of institutional care: the worker as part of the client's social world—bringing in 'outside' news as a quasi-friend or one that brings domestic skills to the maintenance of the client's homespace.

Yet regulatory issues specific to home care shape how the materiality of care practices is actually played out. One homemaker spoke, for example, of the constraints placed on her that prevent her from doing work that she feels is integral to the spirit of care:

> In a house where you have a little old lady living by herself that's full of arthritis . . . if we're not allowed to move the chair that she sits in to get the crumbs underneath, or wipe off the top of the fridge . . . she ends up hiring someone in to do the work I feel we should be doing for them. (homemaker)

Other workers 'bend the rules'; expressions of emotional care were used to rationalize such action. For example, one homemaker interpreted the decision she made as being an integral part of the care needs of the client:

> Like ah, we're not supposed to do windows. But I had a client that all she did was sit and look out the window. So I cleaned the area so she could see out the window. Now that isn't windows, that's ahm, ah, what do you call it, ah, fun time for the client, you know. That's her only [entertainment] . . . because she never went anywhere . . . but she sat looking out the window. So I always kept the window clean for her . . . it was a health issue, as far as I'm concerned, the health of the person. (homemaker)

The quotes in this section of the chapter are suggestive of the varying conditions under which paid care work takes place. They also indicate how the relationship between care worker and care recipient, and the specificity of what constitutes care work, are located within regulatory frameworks and particular locales. The employer may be an agency or, in a few instances, a care recipient using a direct payment scheme. Care workers may be employed by a number of agencies, or a client may be served by more than one agency, which further complicates issues of authority and autonomy in relation to both care worker and care recipient. Other factors, such as continuities or transiency in caregivers also impinge on how the care relationship may be managed.

In the rest of the chapter, we discuss one case example to further unravel the negotiation of care work, its regulation and the care relationship. This closer focus helps us to illustrate the constitution of homespace as care space and to comment on how the complex materialities and social practices of care involved are closely implicated in the production of an ethic of care—one that includes both caring about and caring for.

HOME SPACE AS CARE SPACE: AN ETHIC OF CARE IN PRACTICE

We draw on data from one case to illustrate the interwoven dimensions of care and how these are actively reflected upon and addressed by care workers and family caregivers in their everyday care practices. The case is one where the care recipient, 'Andrew', has complex care needs, and at the time of the study was no longer able to speak (and therefore not able to be interviewed). His adult son lived in the same house and was the primary caregiver. The house was described by one worker as atypical in its particularly poor conditions, although another commented that there were others the same or worse. The nurse, registered practical nurse (RPN) and homemaker were interviewed. Although the care recipient was not able to participate in an interview, we see this case as useful in throwing into sharp relief the non-uniform, and sometimes difficult, conditions under which care is given and the vulnerabilities of both caregivers and receivers.

We look at the negotiation of rules, the emotional work of the care worker/care recipient relationship and the communication between the workers and family caregiver. Such negotiation shows considerable tension between the desire to provide good quality care and the constraints imposed by the particularities of home space and the regulatory framework of home care. The case of Andrew demonstrates the complexity of creating a care space that can meet the conditions of ethical caring. What is achieved is done partly by challenging regulations and bringing a bit 'extra' into the caregiver/care recipient relationship.

Care Work and Emotional Labor

Asked about the rewards of caregiving work in general, Andrew's homemaker stated:

> It's great! You're helping somebody to be self-sufficient . . . there's a lot of vacuuming and scrubbing and stuff like that, but if you put it in—that you're helping somebody to stay in their own home, you know, if you look at it that way it's a worthwhile job, you know.

Her comments were echoed by the RPN and other care workers in the study. Keeping a person with care needs comfortable for as long as possible at home—a place familiar to them and where they, as far as possible, can continue to choose to do things they enjoy when they like and in an environment where they have some control—necessarily creates a relationship between care worker and client that is potentially quite different than might be seen in a hospital or other formal care setting. While a hospital, for example, is laden with power relations visible in the design of its institutional setting, its routinized activities and the assembly of practice personnel, the home as a symbolic site mediates such relations and routines. Its prime association is with the person residing there, often over a long period of time, and its usual location in a neighborhood setting all shape the care worker/client relationship. As the RPN noted, when asked about her relationship with the client, someone to whom she has provided care for several years:

> Ah, it's still provider/client [relationship] but ahm, you know, I guess
> you shouldn't get that involved in—in a situation like that, but it's very
> difficult not to, especially when you're in a home; it's different and you
> see what his life is like. . . . you develop a closeness with them, you
> know. . . . It's not a professional thing to do, but when you're in close
> proximity to someone for that period of time . . . you do get involved in
> their life . . . You can't help but get involved with them.

So while workers valued the need to maintain professionalism on the job,
the intimacy of care and its association with a 'life-in-context' seemed to
bring an additional dimension to how they interpreted and practiced their
work. Of course, emotional attachments can be forged in any care relationship in any setting, but when care is provided in the home, the emotional
labor of care work may be recast. Workers are often working in less than
ideal conditions and in the attempt to create a professionally appropriate
environment that also respects the emotional (caring about) as well as physical (caring for) needs of the client, tensions emerge around the negotiation
of tasks and the regulations circumscribing these. Andrew's case was particularly problematic in terms of its physical safety due to especially unsani-
tary conditions—for both client and care worker. Not only is the client's
body vulnerable in such conditions, but so too is that of the carer.

Workplace Environment as a Place of Risk

The care workers were uniform in their opinion of the workplace conditions
of Andrew's home. One dimension was that of the conditions of the home
itself, which incorporated risk for the care worker in particular, although
potentially also for the client. A second dimension was the rural setting in
which the home was located, which brought problems in creating a safe
environment for care.

The homemaker described how the circumstances of the family caregiver, the client's son, had changed, which had effects on what jobs were
allocated to her:

> The general condition of his home has changed in the last . . . five years
> that I've been going there . . . Now Home Care has taken us out of the
> home to do vacuuming, scrubbing dishes, and cleaning. . . . Our main
> job is, ahm, [the client] himself, his care. Like we make sure he's clean,
> dry, bedding, his room, vacuum, dusting, we just pertain to his room
> now. We used to look after the whole house.

Since this change the cleanliness of the rest of the home has deteriorated,
and the RPN describes her uneasiness in these terms:

> There's garbage everywhere, dirt, the bathroom is filthy, ahm, you
> know, Andrew's room is not bad because the homemakers, ah, you

know, try and keep it clean. But ahm, I hate having to go into any other section of the house.

The nurse similarly points out the poor conditions of the home, although, again, notes the contrast to the client's own room which is the responsibility of the homemaker:

> ... normally there are cases of empty, ahm, ah, the nutritional stuff substance that [the client] takes in through his gastrostomy tube ... a person-high stack of empty cans. [The client's] room itself is kept clean, the homemakers do that, but they're only responsible for the space that he's using.

The RPN commented on the difficulty in preparing medications in such conditions:

> You try and keep the area where you're preparing his meds and his feed like, I have a small area there and you try and keep that area clean because the rest of the counter is just a disaster.

Later in the interview the nurse notes a further complicating factor, that of an uncertain water supply which is from a well. This makes housecleaning and care providing tasks more difficult at certain times of the year. She noted:

> the problem is that because they're on a cistern ... there's often a problem with water availability. You may not have had any rain so therefore you don't have any water, which means that like even something as simple as washing your hands can be difficult, and then somebody says "well I wouldn't want to touch the towels that are in the bathroom anyway." And I usually do wash my hands in the bathroom, but then we also have a hand sanitizer.

Water problems make all the care workers' tasks more difficult. The homemaker recounted:

> the water is not always—they don't have the water to do stuff with, so sometimes, ahm, we don't even have water to bath Andrew. We have to—they have water in a jug and we pour the water in, we have to heat the tea kettle to get warm water sometimes. . . . His well went dry because the position that they're in, the wells went dry so we had special stuff for sterilizing our hands so we don't have to wash them. Because they had the water tested and there was a bacteria in the water so we had to use sterilization.

There is a clear potential for health hazards in working in poor conditions. In this case, the RPN spoke of the fear of infection due to the dirtiness of the home and commented on the odors from garbage that had not been disposed of. In other cases, smoking can be problem for a care worker, as well as instances of pulled muscles through lifting heavy clients. In the case discussed here, the main problems primarily concerned hygiene.

NEGOTIATING RISK

In order to manage these conditions and problems with water supply, care workers talked of the bedroom of the client as a relatively safe, clean environment. Nevertheless, care workers had to 'bend' the rules in order to achieve a satisfactory standard for providing the care. As the homemaker said:

> as a homemaker my first instinct is to clean the bathroom totally, but we've been told no. Andrew is our care, and we have to shut our eyes to the other, if that's how they want to live, and that's how they want to live. But every once in a while I'll clean that sink up and the taps.

The RPN also spoke of the homemaker's role in keeping a level of cleanliness in parts of the house which the care workers need to use, but Andrew does not:

> Like you can't wash your hands in the bathroom because the towels are so dirty. . . . We counted one time; three and a half months before the towel was taken down. And only because the homemaker took it and washed it, you know. And actually her responsibility is not that part of the house; it's only for Andrew's stuff. She does all his laundry, his towels, his sheets, his gown, all his stuff. But she couldn't stand it anymore. She took the towel and washed it.

But perhaps a bigger issue is the water supply, and here all the care workers are put in the position of bringing water in. The nurse carries a jug of water in her car as a matter of course. The homemaker says they each bring a jug of water from their own homes for the client's use—for preparing his medication and feeds—during the month of August when the well water is low. It is stored in the kitchen, so the kitchen needs to be used even though it is off-bounds for cleaning by the homemaker. All the care workers routinely carry antiseptic hand cleanser to avoid using the facilities in the house.

TEAMWORK AND BOUNDARY CROSSINGS

Teamwork was part of the picture of creating an environment suitable for providing appropriate physical care for Andrew. This was not prescribed team work, but a matter of the care workers informally negotiating tasks. Cleanliness, for example, was facilitated by the homemaker using her own initiative to wash a bathroom towel. The handling of soiled bed linen was another task where care workers had to make decisions about the bounds of their work. The RPN talked of having to wash out particularly badly soiled linen, rather than putting it in the laundry basket. She would bring water into Andrew's room and wash it in a basin there, as it was not possible to do it in the bathroom or kitchen. She would then let the homemaker know and she would launder it. A communication book was the main way of communicating among the different care workers. Occasionally the care workers may meet each other on the way in or out of the home, in which case they may discuss the client briefly.

The family caregiver, the son of the client, was incorporated into how tasks were handled. Despite complaints about his poor housecleaning the care workers made an effort to get along with him. The RPN noted that the son would help her move the client, for example when she was suffering from an elbow injury, and would also pick up things the caregivers need. He also monitored the medical equipment and alerted the RPN or nurse if there seemed to be a problem. Structurally, the relationship between care workers and family caregiver is an ambiguous one: all are concerned with the client's care but each is located differently in a moral field that contextualizes how a professional relationship is enacted, together with particular expectations of what 'care' entails. Spatially it may also be fraught with tension, especially in this case where the carespace within the home is surrounded by the homespace of the son—with different notions of how this should or can be maintained.

Quality of Care?

Despite the various difficulties in working in this home, the care workers were unanimous in believing the client was receiving good care. While this was defined in terms of 'set up' and Andrew's ability to remain at home, so focusing on the physical, practical dimensions of care, there was also clearly an emotional side to the ways in which care was provided. This related not only to aspects of the hands-on body work but also to the 'extras' that were given. For instance, there was evidence that care workers continued to converse with the client despite his loss of speech. The nurse said, "I always put in a little gab here and there either to get a smile out of him or . . . just some kinda response." But the extras were sometimes technically outside the rules. Commonly, care workers would phone in to let the agency know they were planning to do something 'extra' and get approval, but other times this was not deemed necessary.

The care workers were well aware of regulations concerning what care and services could be provided, knowing also that they were not allowed to receive gifts or money from clients and must keep the relationship on a business level. However, as noted earlier, it is hard for care workers not to have some emotional involvement with client and family caregivers. There is a blurring between gifts and being considerate and concerned for someone, which we can see to different extents. The context also makes a difference. For example, the nurse will go out of her way more for palliative care patients and will pick up medications or pharmacy items on her own time, particularly if the client or family members have difficulty doing this. Other expressions of care took the form of a more conventional gift, although without monetary value. A clear distinction is also made between the blurred area of gifting and other rules. For example, the homemaker said:

> If I have [vegetables in the garden] I bring some stuff in for them. That's about it. . .. 'Cause I try to keep it on a business level, because it's not, ah, (sigh) if you—if you take it past the professional, you're the professional in the home so if you take things personal, which is very hard not to do, but I try to keep it at a business level.
>
> *Interviewer:* And why do you do that?
>
> *Homemaker:* Because of my job and that's what we're told to do. I mean, ah, I suppose I could lend a little bit more help like ah, you know, (but) what we're not allowed to do is (not always clear) if he [client's son] wanted to go to town and it's raining, could I give him a ride into town or could I loan him my car, I don't do that. And he doesn't ask.

The capacity to give 'an extra thought' can be seen as texturing a care relationship in ways not envisaged in the formal concept of care assumed by regulations and rules, based on the notion of caring for without the dimension of caring about. While there is insufficient data in this study to do more than speculate, it seems it may be the care workers in the less-skilled sector of care work, essentially transferring domestic labor skills from their home to another's, who find this type of gifting more compatible with a homemaking care mandate than for those providing nursing or other health professional skills.

DISCUSSION: MATERIALIZING CARE

The empirical material here illustrates that the everyday practices of care that bring together caring for and caring about are the mode through which care is 'materialized'. In our study the homes of care recipients simultaneously are workplaces for caregivers. They are also at a point of articulation of local and wider processes which, in a range of larger scales or contextual features, shape how the home is brought into being as a care space. These include national economies, regional restructuring of care provision and the specific homes and neighborhoods that provide the physical site of the actual care. Some care workers are international migrants, falling at the bottom of a hierarchy of care work, so also bringing in global processes into the home of care receivers (Datta et al. 2010; England and Dyck, 2011b).

The data show the complex negotiation of care work as workers interpret and put into practice agency rules about eligible tasks and manage the affective as well as the corporeal dimensions of the care relation. The dual vulnerability of care workers and care recipients is evident—but in different ways. Vulnerability can relate to material bodies, a social self or valued identity. The vulnerable body and social 'self' of the care recipient is an area where both a professional relationship on the part of the care worker and the affective dimension of the relationship come into play. Quasi-friendships or detached professionalism result in different experiences of the care relationship and may create different climates in which an ethic of care may flourish. Care workers are also vulnerable. Their bodies are vulnerable when doing heavy work or working in conditions that generally could be considered unhealthy (smoky, cluttered or dirty environments). As a low-paid member of a workforce with little security, they are also vulnerable to marketplace forces and are administered from a distance through labor regulations and agencies' rules. While such regulations are in place ostensibly to protect the worker, they also bring areas of ambiguity that can place the worker's job at risk.

It was noted at the start of the chapter that the care relation is inflected by both power and affect or emotion. One aspect of this power is realized through the specific relationship of a worker/care recipient. But power also enters the care relation through practices and procedures emanating from beyond the care site—in the policies and regulations devised to shape the meaning given to 'community care' and put into practice by those working for agencies working within those policies and regulations. As Foucault famously stated, there is always potential for resistance where there is power. In negotiating rules, workers in effect are resisting power in Foucauldian terms. But this may come with a penalty. There is little space for the emotional dimension of care work in the labyrinth of regulatory mechanisms, and considerable ambiguity in the interpretation of some acts of care. A small kindness outside the bounds of eligible tasks can, for example, lead to dismissal. If a worker is in the dilemma of the care worker who noted the contradiction between providing care and not being allowed to carry water, then how is an ethic of care to be realized? Body work and the workspaces of the home are 'invisible' yet regulated through rules and procedures. While one care worker (as above) phones in to check before doing a task about which she is not sure, others do not. The invisiblized space of the home as a paid work site is both a benefit and a negative in its ambiguity. At best it is a way for those most vulnerable in society to continue living and ageing in a dignified and respectful way, with needs responded to as required, at worst a replication of rigid bureaucracy, exploitation of workers and lack of control for those with perhaps little remaining in most areas of their lives.

The identification of care needs and the responsibility for provision of these is enacted through care agencies, although the circumscribing of eligible tasks and employment conditions of care workers (such as 'casual labor' contracts, low pay and regulations that hinder their definition of quality care) affect the level of quality of care. These care workers certainly can provide competent care, in the sense of appropriate body work for clients, but it is through going beyond what is prescribed that the initial care tasks can be translated into care that meets emotional and social needs of clients, as well as simply physical care. Workplace conditions (of the home) may also compromise the safety of the worker. The vulnerabilities emerging in the study reported here suggest there is the potential for the care of the client and the safety of the worker to fall beneath acceptable standards in such hidden spaces, although in this study there was no evidence of this. It was through professionalism, and careful negotiation of homespaces and clients' needs, that on a personal, case-by-case level, clients received high-quality care. It is at the point of institutional and regional organization that an ethic of care needs to be comprehensively explored—what rules and mechanisms promote or inhibit its enactment?

An ethic of care needs to be inclusive of both carers and care recipients. There also needs to be awareness of intersections of gender, class and 'race' in understanding the mechanisms of power in emotionally laden labor with the need of a rich vein of work in tracing such intersectionality to fully comprehend the power and affective dimensions of care work and how these are materialized through different scales. International comparison is also important if we are to get away from addressing the home as merely a local site for care—a commonsense way to provide for the vulnerable. That 'local site' is far from local, in that the practices taking place there are shaped by layers of decision-making and processes at different scales. What 'best practices' can be generated at what levels of government, local community and user involvement? How can we ensure that power and emotion-laded relation is materialized in ways that emulate an ethic of care that respects the dignity and needs of both parties to the dyad? These questions need to be at the center of policy development and practice.

NOTES

1. The research team was led by Principal Investigator Patricia McKeever, Faculty of Nursing, University of Toronto. Funding was provided by the Social Sciences and Humanities Research Council of Canada. The names of the participants are pseudonyms.

REFERENCES

Armstrong, Patricia and Hugh Armstrong. 2003. *Wasting away: The undermining of Canadian health care.* 2nd ed. Oxford University Press: Toronto.

Aronson, Jane and Sheila Neysmith. 1997. The retreat of the state and long-term care provision: implications for frail elderly people, unpaid family carers and paid home care workers. *Studies in Political Economy* 53: 37–65.

Barnett, Clive. 2005. Who cares? In *Introducing human geographies*, 2nd ed., edited by Phillip Crang, Paul Cloke, and Mark Goodwin, 588–601. London: Arnold.

Bondi, Liz. 2008. On the relational dynamics of caring: a psychotherapeutic approach to emotional and power dimensions of women's care work. *Gender, Place & Culture* 15(3): 249–265.

Datta, Kavita, Cathy McIlwaine, Yara Evans, Joanne Herbert, Jon May and Jane Wills. 2010. A migrant ethic of care? negotiating care and caring among migrant workers in London's low pay economy. *Feminist Review* 94: 93–116.

Dyck, Isabel, Pia Kontos, Jan Angus and Patricia McKeever. 2005. The home as a site for long-term care: meanings and management of bodies and spaces. *Health and Place* 11: 173–185.

England, Kim and Isabel Dyck. 2011a. Managing the body work of home care. *Sociology of Health and Illness* 33(2): 206–219.

—— 2011b. Migrant workers in home care: Responsibilities, routes and respect. (unpublished paper available from the authors).

England, Kim, Joan Eakin, Denise Gastaldo and Patricia McKeever. 2007. Neoliberalizing home care: Managed competition and restructuring home care in Ontario. In *Neoliberalization: Networks, states, peoples*, edited by Kim England and Kevin Ward, 169–194. Blackwell/Antipode: Oxford.

Fisher, Berenice and Joan Tronto. 1990. Towards a feminist theory of caring. In *Circles of care, work and identity in women's lives*, edited by Emily Abel and Margaret Nelson, 35–62. Albany: State University of New York Press.

Healey, Stephen. 2008. Caring for ethics and the politics of health care reform in the United States. *Gender, Place and Culture* 15(3): 267–284.

McKeever, Patricia, Helen Scott, Mary Chipman, Kathy Osterlund and Joan Eakin. 2006. 'Hitting Home': a survey of housing conditions of homes used for long term care in Ontario, Canada. *International Journal of Health Services* 36(3): 521–533.

Mol, Annemarie. 2008. *The logic of care: Health and the problem of patient choice*. London: Routledge.

Nettleton, Sarah and Roger Burrows. 1994. From bodies in hospitals to people in the community: a theoretical analysis of the relocation of health care. *Care in Place* 1: 93–103.

Tronto, Joan 1993. *Moral boundaries: A political argument for an ethic of care*. New York: Routledge.

Part II

Care

4 'To Work Out What Works Best'
What is Good in Home Care?

Christine Ceci

Most western, industrialized societies have developed systems for providing homemaking and health-related supports to older people who require assistance to continue to live in their own homes (Purkis, Ceci and Björnsdottir 2008). In our present context, one increasingly framed by concern for the challenges presented by ageing populations, the appropriate, feasible and acceptable parameters of home care have been much discussed, particularly the contribution the home care sector must make to ensure the sustainable future of the Canadian health system (Baranek, Deber and Williams 2004; Ceci and Purkis 2011; Coyte and McKeever 2001; Duncan and Reutter 2006; Pringle 2006; Romanow 2002). Yet home care, as a formal practice, remains significantly under-theorized. Though expected to do much—from managing clients with complex medical needs to supporting frail or chronically ill persons—many of the concrete elements and everyday realities that constitute this practice and site of care remain largely unexamined. So although Canada is a leader in important aspects of home care research, with investigations ranging from economic implications (Aronson and Neysmith 2006), cost effectiveness (Hollander and Chappell 2002, 2003), appropriate delivery systems (Hollander and Prince 2007) and the gendered politics of home care (Flood 1999; Gregor 1997) to the recent contributions of human geography (Andrews 2003; Angus et al. 2005), there has been less attention to the micro contexts of home care, the level at which care is created and experienced (Twigg 2006).

This means, for example, that while those responsible for managing home care are responding to pressures to increase the efficiency of the system, this is being done with little knowledge of what is actually essential to providing good care (Purkis, Ceci and Björnsdottir 2008). This, then, is the too-large but necessary focus for this paper: what *is* good care in home care? Or more specifically—for it is the nature of care as such to be specific—for older people who require supportive care or services to continue to live in their own homes, what does help look like and how may it be best accomplished? I pose this as a question even though I know it is too large and in some respects not answerable, or rather, it is the sort of question that in its specifics will have many answers. Nevertheless it seems to me that if we had a clearer sense of what *kind* of care is called for in home care, what kind of care responds best to the conditions of life encountered here, we might have a better sense of what to do, of which practices to support and which to resist—and importantly, what other questions we should be asking.

Certainly in the 'micro' contexts of care—the everyday enactments of practices of home care—questions of what constitutes 'good care' matter enormously. For example, in my own research[1] I have noted 'points of worry' that seem to arise from difficulties in enacting what might recognizably be called 'good care'—as hazy a concept as that is—including gaps between the supports and services offered to people and what they actually seem to need (Ceci 2006a), tensions related to the availability and use of risk discourses alongside the difficulties of acting on assessed risks (Ceci and Purkis 2009; Purkis 2001), professional care providers who find their work increasingly meaningless (Ceci 2006b), and organizational practices that have trouble responding to the 'human-ness' of the work (Ceci 2008). These and other similar points of worry seem to arise from a growing reliance on a kind of proceduralism in the organization of care practices, a bureaucratic rationality that responds to, and is the effect of, mounting societal anxiety concerning the (apparently) increasing demands of older people and the economic 'realities' that will (apparently) preclude their fulfillment. Such a rationality is not neutral, containing as it does its own, often silent, normative intention, a normativity, it must be noted, more associated with managing rather than meeting people's needs. Though such proceduralism in the organization of practices may have its own 'goods', such as efficiency or predictability, these are not necessarily responsive or appropriate to the matter of concern of home care practices, that is, the question of how people are going to be able to live their lives. For people who are older, perhaps frail, and requiring mainly supportive types of assistance to continue to live 'independently', the logic of 'good' practice, its intentionality, will need to respond satisfactorily to the question of how to help when it is a matter of how one is going to be able to live daily life, rather than the more usual healthcare question of how to 'get well' or be cured (Struhkamp, Mol and Swierstra 2008). And, at the very least, it seems reasonable to suggest that we are looking for more than arrangements that must merely be endured.

In this paper I want to try to clarify this question of the intentionality of home care practice, and to do this I draw on observations of the practices of home care case managers, as well as conversations with them about these practices, collected during a field study of home care in a mid-size western Canadian city. In Canada, home care programs are conceptualized and delivered through provincial authorities, sometimes further devolved to regional levels, leading to a patchwork of supports and services across the country that reflects both locally available resources and prevailing ideologies. Though there is some federal influence exerted through transfer payments to the provinces, home care services are bound by neither federal legislation nor national standards, and although most provinces fund some components of home care, local policy makers determined local practices of cost sharing and service levels. Care is not an entitlement and access, depending on the cost-sharing arrangements in place, may be linked to ability to pay. In general, the further one moves from traditionally conceived health or medical services, and from professional to non-professional services, the more attenuated are the arguments for public provision of services.

As well as the empirical resources developed from this fieldwork, I also draw on Michel Foucault's thinking about the nature of practices, particularly his observation that "'practices' don't exist without a certain regime of rationality" (1991, 79). Or as Burchell, Gordon and Miller note, Foucault's insistence that even the crassest and most obtuse parts of social reality contain a "parcel of thought" and that creating visibility around this intentionality, putting this thought into words, first, deprives it of its self-evidence and, second, assists in making the practice of concern thinkable and thus changeable (1991, ix–x). For Foucault, practices possess their own 'reason'; they are inscribed by forms of rationality, codes of knowledge and rules of conduct that shape their intelligibility and acceptability, and, at the same time, form their principles and strategies of justification (1991, 75–79). Mol (2008) also draws attention to the logic of practices. Like Foucault, Mol does not use this term to refer to either logic as philosophy or to logical-ness in the ordinary sense of a mode of reasoning, but rather to underline that intelligibility or coherence are implicit or embedded in practices, practices have a sense or intention, and that bringing this to language helps us to talk about it. Logic, she writes, "is meant to evoke the sense that locally, some things are more comprehensible than others" (8). And as she and Foucault both suggest, articulating the logic of practices allows us to raise and explore questions of what is understood as appropriate, fitting and even desirable to do in a particular site, and what is not.

This attention to the logic of practices makes sense if we accept Mol's argument that good care is not an ideal but a practice. She writes, "'good care' is not an ideal that can be defended in general terms, as a matter of principle. . . . Instead it is something that people shape, invent and adapt, time and again, in everyday practices" (2008, 4).[2] Care of all sorts is constituted through practices that are complex, heterogeneous and frequently ambiguous in terms of their effects. But perhaps it is in terms of the effects of practices that we may best read intentionality. If, as Mol suggests, good care begins with working out, in practices, what will work best in specific situations, then better or worse practices and indeed the nature of good care itself will depend, in part, on what we wish to accomplish. Or as Moser writes, "in this process, what counts is what works, and works for the better, and so makes an improvement in the specific everyday relations in which the patient is placed" (2010, 293). Already we begin to see that although good care may not have a pre-specified content, it may have a distinctive character. In the idea of working out what works best, practice informed by a logic of care takes on an ethos of specificity, iteration, constant improvement; practices we would support would be those that can enact this variability, flexibility and responsiveness. And we could resist those that refuse this. That is, by articulating the logic of current home care practices, we may begin to see the *kinds* of practices, questions and possibilities that respond best to what matters—when what matters is how to live *with* frailty or a chronic condition.

As may be clear, this sort of analysis requires specific knowledge of the practices of concern in order to develop a sense of what is appropriate, needed or satisfactory in a particular situation (Mol 2008). Like Mol, I turn to data obtained through fieldwork in the ethnographic mode to reflect on the logic that informs the practices of home care as enacted through the work and words of home care case managers. Over many months, I shadowed home care case managers[3] as they went about their work, first, to gain an understanding of the conditions shaping their field of practice and second, to learn what help looks like in this setting, to see how care for older people is crafted through the practices of formal care providers such as case managers (Ceci 2006a, 2006b, 2008; Ceci and Purkis 2009). In Mol's case, she examined the practices associated with treatment of and life with diabetes in a medium-sized Dutch town. Though this may seem an incongruous point of reference for a study of home care in Canada, Mol's helpful direction here is her analysis of the intentionality of a set of practices rather than an elaboration of their specific content—though this is there as well. However, for me, of significance is her meticulous and detailed comparison of practices informed by the logic of care with those informed by a logic of choice, contrasting, even competing, rationalities that are nonetheless both enacted in practices in this setting. She chose to explore this problematic in part because the ideal of patient choice, generally assumed to be an undeniably good thing, is more and more drawn into the practices of health care in 'the West'; the logic of choice alters daily practice in significant ways yet may not improve 'care' or serve patients all that well, particularly those whose need is to live with a condition or disease rather than be cured of it. Mol is careful to differentiate her doubts about choice as a fitting logic of practice from those who argue that the important questions about choice concern whether or not people are actually able to make choices. Instead of being concerned with the abilities of people in this way, she directs our attention to the practices in which people are involved. For example, in considering not only moments of choosing but "situations of choice," we see that in living a life with a disease, people are engaged in many practical activities among which episodic moments of choosing may not actually have central significance (Mol 2008, 7). Further, our different capacities to engage in any of these activities, including the activity of making choices, may not rest 'in' us but with the ordering of the situation (see also Moser 2005).

Mol's (2008) analytical shift from individual capacities to situations of choice or care resonated very strongly for me and with my observations in the field of home care where encounters between case managers and clients seemed to constitute events organized around the problem of frailty, but in which the solutions crafted through practices often seemed as fragile as the people requiring care. This is probably not surprising, as good intentions and local arrangements are increasingly fragmented in the face of budget 'realities' and distant system issues, rather than shaped by responsiveness to what people might actually need. In fact, the significant pressures on home care resources seem to have resulted in a narrowing of vision, the range of recognized needs all the time more constrained by the perceived ability to respond (Ceci 2008). At the same time, unplanned consequences of distal management strategies create new types of home care clients on an *ad hoc* basis through policies and practices that, for example, decrease the absolute number of institutional beds available, that discharge people from hospital 'sicker and quicker' or that narrow the eligibility requirements for home care programs. One effect of these sorts of practices is to transfer the acuity traditionally associated with institutional settings to home environments and in so doing to institute competition for 'scarce' resources between the newer, more acute and medically fragile clients and the traditional clients of home care, those who are older and frail (Purkis 2001). The index case of who is to be considered an appropriate user of home care resources shifts upward in relation to medically defined acuity and the legitimacy of need, and the problem of frailty, is reconfigured. But for all that these effects of constrained resources, prioritized medical need and shifting services are not surprising, especially amid fears of the unsustainability of the health system, there remains the *situation* of the 'traditional' clients of home care, situations that become increasingly unlivable through the inadequacies of care. It is the situation of these persons that is of concern here and I take my cue and my question once again from Foucault: "since there is this suffering, and since there are these practices and this kind of knowledge and these kinds of institutions which are supposed to effect a cure, are they really doing something" (1989, 418)?

So following Mol's (2008) lead, I treat the data of my fieldwork[4] as a case study through which I may draw out the logics of observed practices, particularly those of care and choice, consider what practices actually seem to be helping people and, through this, try to develop a sense of what we might be working toward in this field of care. It is important to note here that Mol makes no claims as to the general applicability of her analysis. She does not even claim that the logic of care is always intrinsically better. Rather, it is her position that it simply deserves to be better attended to (2008, 79). Mol's analysis sets out a problematic for health care in general, asking whether it is possible to articulate a logic of care that gives words to what 'good care' is about (84). Responding to this question in the specific context of home care seems to me something worth attempting and the analysis that follows involves an examination of the mix of logics apparent in this setting: the bureaucratic proceduralism demanded by organizational priorities, the boundaries of responsibility set out through the logic of choice, the responsiveness of practices informed by care, and the risks of neglect when care is overlooked.

CONDITIONS OF PRACTICE: ORGANIZATIONAL PRIORITIES

Home care, as a system, enacts many assumptions about what it is that older people need. Currently, and of course arguably, a good deal of how these assumptions are materialized and enacted in practices seems related less to what older people might actually need and more to the (necessary) demands of organization and order, demands that it appears are thought to be best handled, or at least most effectively managed, if they are worked out in advance. As Bauman writes, "order-making tends to be, as a rule, undertaken in the name of fighting chaos" (2002, 287). In home care, this feared chaos becomes visible in the growing tendency, evident in many western nations, to conceptualize home care as a sector of health care imminently in danger of being swamped by the grey wave of an ageing population. Based in what some have described as an "apocalyptic demography," older people as a group are viewed as "a time bomb that [will] sooner or later damage society"—primarily due to the rising costs of their care (Rozanova, Northcott, and McDaniel 2006, 381–384). The specter of unrelenting demand for increasingly scarce and costly resources is reinforced in myriad everyday home care practices and settings. For example, in fieldnotes recorded during long-term care program meetings, the largest part of the data concerned frequent discussions about the need to more efficiently manage demand for care in order to meet budget goals, primarily through actions such as eliminating certain kinds of clients from eligibility for care or re-conceptualizing some types of services as now unnecessary. Sometimes ignored, sometimes explicitly acknowledged, was the fact that these actions were being undertaken not because people's needs had changed but because there were simply not enough 'hours' to go around (Christine Ceci, fieldnotes). Case managers' questions about the impact of service cuts on their particular clients were deflected by a reorientation to larger budget realities and their manager's rational, rationalizing argument that there was a "need to start somewhere . . . there are more complex clients in the community and more of them . . . there are finite resources and these need to be put to the greater needs" (Ceci, fieldnotes). Potentially overwhelming demand requires a narrow and disciplined focus, one which needs to work to curtail the claims of those at the periphery—claims that may only arise in close encounters between case managers and older people—through a centralized control of practices (Law 1994).

Yet this apparently sensible, understandable impulse to create order, to forestall chaos, to manage events so that at least some form of care may be offered to some people may have effects that are not especially helpful. One of the dangers in the elaboration and securing of any particular ordering, and perhaps a danger not entirely avoidable, is that any ordering intention assumes, and subdues, only its particular chaos. As Bauman continues, "there would be no chaos were there no ordering intention already in place and were not the 'regular situation' already conceived in advance so that its promotion could start in earnest" (2002, 287). Bauman draws our attention to the ways that fore-understandings order practices, including working to position what is outside of a particular ordering, such as alternative practice arrangements, as part of the chaos to be avoided. This suggests that our (limited) sense of what should be the case, of how, for instance, a system should manage expectations and people, works to form an advance intention linked only to the particular chaos—excessive demand for services—that practices then seek to avoid. In home care, current practices, or the 'regular situation' to be accomplished, revolve around a question of how to best *manage* people's needs, how to hold back uncontrolled demand, and the organization's central ambitions, to be effective and efficient in this, are clearly appropriate to these managerial ends. Whether a system formed through this intentionality is able to meet as well as manage people's needs is another question altogether.

This makes the reality currently enacted in many home care practice settings a predominantly bureaucratic one, with its prevailing logic oriented to this managing of older people's needs. In meetings between case managers and program managers, in conversations between case managers and clients and in organizational documents, managerial priorities are made visible and their specific reality built up through a preoccupation with forms, billing strategies, time-task calculations, algorithms that assign care levels and other new data collection practices. These work to create the kind of measurable reality that is most amenable to bureaucratic tactics, that is, to being managed through quantitative calculations—cutting back the number of eligible service hours for the different care levels, reducing the number of minutes allocated for particular tasks, subtracting whole categories of clients from eligibility for care. In an interview, a senior program manager's justification for the withdrawal of care from clients with so-called lower level care needs[5] reflects the authority and sense of inevitability associated with this form of practice:

> . . . *that* particular direction came from the ministry, in terms of where we needed to put our resources. [They] did not give any additional resources to home and community care, and because we were taking on more and more clients, that meant we either had to water down the resources to everybody, or reduce services to those at the lighter care level. (Ceci, key informant interview)

Managers must address the budget realities that are handed down to them and one way they do so is by transferring this concern to case managers, who then take this prioritizing practice to clients. In the words of another manager, her role was to "educate the [case managers], and help them deal with that reduction in resource, for them to be able to do their work . . . and to pass the information on to clients appropriately" and interestingly, she went on, "to still help with the client's plan" (Ceci, key informant interview).

New priorities are also written into the documents intended to guide practice. In an interview, yet another program manager explained, "I've just revised the home support section of our staff manual and there's just budget written all over it. . . . I mean it talks about client needs, but the overall or underlying or whatever you want to call it, is budget" (Ceci, key informant interview). Each link builds up the budget as the intractable 'fact' to be dealt with, an indisputable kind of 'reality' that is increasingly offered as the justification for how one practices until we finally have a case manager describing her intention to limit her involvement with clients because "the budget was just in such tough shape" (Ceci, fieldnotes). The practices in place secure the reality most able to respond to the worrying scenario of unchecked demand; they bring the care available to people in line with budget 'realities'. The logic of practices here shifts the focus from older people as particular persons with specific needs to the ways in which these (assessed) needs may be best managed, that is, aligned with organizational capacity.

Yet even here, in a context where the overriding logic is directed to managing the potentially unmanageable, it is possible to observe friction in the logics that drive practices, for instance when case managers attempt to advance their more immediate, personal experiences with clients as *also* a reasonable ground for making decisions about how to proceed. However, their talk of practices of advocacy, of feeling personal responsibility to particular clients or shaping services to meet individual needs tends to be crowded out by an economic rationality oriented to "living within our means" and "focusing on essentials" (Ceci, fieldnotes). And this is a rationality almost impossible to deny. Those who manage the case managers' work urge them instead to be resourceful and creative, to do more with less, and to use their professional judgment in assessing situations to determine which of their many clients can be said to have the greatest need. At the same time, and perhaps paradoxically, their capacities to act on their professional judgments, capacities for discretion they are understood to develop through their interactions with people, are increasingly dispersed across the guidelines and forms that (pre)-organize their practices. This reality, rather than one openly oriented to questions of how to best support people who are living with frailty, structures the possibilities of case managers' performance, and it is pulled through to their engagements with people. At the center of home care then, is an essential proceduralism intended to manage older people's needs, to keep people and their needs in line with the present estimation of the possible. Case managers' practices are constituted through this rationality and from here they are sent out into 'the world' to find out how to help people—but again paradoxically, from within an organizational context that in so many words and practices, tells them not to.

Given this overwhelming and, for some, irresistible organizational and societal anxiety concerning the increasing demands of older people and the economic 'realities' that preclude their fulfillment, it seems fair to take a moment and consider whether questions about the nature of good care for older people are reasonable ones to ask, or whether these sorts of questions miss the point that we *really* have no choices here. At this point, I will just observe that this is a political question and part of what makes it a political question is the idea that if reality emerges through and is enacted in practices, then reality is, like practices, multiple, complex and changing (Mol 2008; Moser 2006). As Moser writes, "if realities are practiced and multiple rather than singular and given . . . they bring up the question of what reality we want to live with and what reality to realize" (543). Organizational practices and the bureaucratic logic that currently dominates them have effects in establishing the patterns of the reality case managers work within and, to some extent, that clients live within. However, any reality is constituted by multiple ordering practices, so other orderings, other logics, will also be at work (Law 1994). As Mol (2008) observes, no practice is 'pure', different sorts of activities and intentions overlap and interfere with one another. Some of these may co-exist harmoniously, some will not (Moser 2005). But for Mol, the important point is that "different logics push and pull in different directions. They turn us into something different" (79). From this perspective, articulating what is at stake in different practices, attending to what these practices turn us into, opens them and us up to question. Attunement to the difficulties of budgets and larger economic conditions, then, does not remove the possibility of providing good care, that is, care that is responsive to what older people need. However, these are conditions that contribute to and partly explain the intelligibility and acceptability of practices that in another context might be seen as intolerable.

LOGICS THAT PUSH AND PULL (1)

To continue the elaboration of this problematic, I look to the practices of case managers who, through their practices, work both for and against this prevailing logic. A way into this question is to ask simply, what happens? What happens when older people who need help connect with the system organized to provide it? I think it is fair to say that many case managers attempt to start from what people say they need, from or with an idea of practice that sees itself as attentive, responsive and at least aware of the unpredictability of daily life. For instance, I often observed case managers who, after collecting their assessment data, filling out their forms and making their calculations, set these aside and asked their clients a question that, oddly enough, seemed unrelated, or in some sense parallel, to these other activities. They would ask what would help, what would be ideal, what can we do (Ceci, fieldnotes)? The case managers' instrumental activities worked to set out certain boundaries, the boundaries of organizational practices, but this other question to clients—what would help?—is one that suggests a rich and supple starting point, one from which case managers and clients might work together to actively determine how to best improve the situation. Here practice is not merely a transaction based on a calculation of need and eligibility for services but a process. In the words of one case manager after a home visit to establish contact with an elderly couple struggling with the unpredictability of the husband's transient ischemic attacks, "successful depends on whether she is comfortable to call me when she needs something. It's a step in a process, for some it's a long process. She's on a journey trying to figure out how to cope" (Ceci, fieldnotes). In Mol's (2008) terms, practices that enabled this case manager to accompany this couple on their journey, that supported them in figuring out together what could be done, would be those that tended towards enacting a logic of care. The 'facts' are collected, the numbers calculated, yes, but what is to be done is not given directly from them—it is yet to be determined. In the logic of care, categories and care levels are merely tools that may or may not help in figuring out what is to be done (Mol 2008), and the 'goods' relevant to this bureaucratic logic, such as accountability and efficiency, are only good in their proper place. Outside their proper place, in trying to live daily life with frailty, they may not be particularly helpful.

But even in this particular case, with a case manager open and asking what would help, the possibilities for such help had already been too rigorously delimited. The problem is the unpredictability of events, but all the proposed solutions seem to need to be scheduled in advance, leading Elizabeth, the client's wife, to observe, "the things one really needs are not available" (Ceci, fieldnotes). In her case what she needs is someone to help with "spot trouble"—the falls, the heavy lifting and other irregular occurrences that characterize her life with a husband subject to transiently incapacitating symptoms, what they understatedly described as "the wobblies." The wobblies stand for the unpredictability of life with frailty, and some of the tensions I observed in case managers' practices arose from bumping up against their limited capacity to respond to what is unexpected in daily life. A good part of this is, again, probably unavoidable, but a question for home care is whether the unpredictability of daily life is best responded to through the increasing tendency towards standardization observed in the current organizational context. This context wants clear limits, measurable outcomes and predictable resource allocations. This couple needs someone to help with "spot trouble." This is not something this case manager can help with.

Which is not to say that this is always the case. Sometimes helping people seems relatively uncomplicated. For example, a quick home visit enabled a very frail older woman and her daughter to successfully negotiate a small increase in their home support hours, one more visit from a home support worker on days when the daughter could not be available. When I asked the case manager how she thought the visit had gone, she told me with evident relief, "it's nice not to have to say no. I look at someone like Mrs. Kent, she's pretty frail, and it seems like not a lot of service to help them keep it together" (Ceci, fieldnotes). For both case manager and client, this was a good visit—what would help was also what was organizationally possible. Her more usual experience, this case manager continued, was having to explain to people how "the system actually works," which is often an explanation of the difference between what they are allowed and what they might need. In this case, though, "the system," the case manager's practice model and the client's needs fit well together—the case manager was able to help, she did not have to say no. This simple encounter however, represents an ideal of case management practice—case manager and client working together towards shared goals, and each aware of and accepting the possibilities and limitations of the situation. This is a model of the practice of home care that when realized enables practice to unfold smoothly and efficiently. As another case manager described it:

> You can ask them what their goal is, and how any resources that you can provide can help them meet that goal and reduce their risk, that kind of thing. . . . You have a meeting of the minds . . . you discuss things, you come up with a plan . . . and you set the plan in place and things sort of happen as you would expect them to. (Ceci, case manager interview)

Assessments are made, eligibility calculated, needed services are identified and offered, agreement is reached and a plan is set into place. What could be simpler—except that things do not always unfold as they should. It is notable that the idea, or ideal, of practice described by this case manager was by way of contrast to her actual practice with a client who resisted her attempts to provide support or to put a plan of care in place. In this case, trouble arose because the client, Eleanor, though elderly and with a long history of a degenerative neurological disease, did not see herself as frail or needing help, or at least not the kind of help the case manager had to offer. As the case manager reported, even when she did convince Eleanor to accept home support, she would have the support workers off "getting fresh fish so she could have *Sole Amandine* for dinner" instead of helping with personal care (Ceci, case manager interview). For the case manager, whose contact was ongoing despite the difficulty of ensuring what she thought of as appropriate support, the challenge came from "trying to provide services for her that you could see she needed, but that she just didn't have the insight to understand." The case manager struggled to "get a handle on what was dementia, what was just her personality and being difficult." There was some agreement among those involved with Eleanor, including her distant family, that she was not "really competent" but, at the same time, she'd also been able to live more or less independently for the two years this case manager had been visiting her. As the case manager said, "she's not really capable of making decisions that are appropriate, but she can do some things and . . . the proof is in the pudding. She's been there, it's been well over two years since I've known her, and there she still is!" When asked, the case manager described her main concerns as being declining attention to personal hygiene, poor housekeeping as well as some socially embarrassing behaviors. "It's tricky," she told me, "because you really do see her failing and living in a way that she would be horrified if she really understood." She described her role as trying to support the home support workers who were visiting Eleanor, trying to maintain her safety and reduce possibilities for harm, and also to advocate for her when complaints arose from other tenants in her building, or from the police or ambulance personnel whom Eleanor tended to call when she ran into any kind of trouble. But because of her ongoing concerns, the case manager had recently decided she would gradually withdraw some of the supports she had managed to put in place, for example the home support subsidy, with the hope that the Eleanor would see that what she really needed was to be in a care facility. In her words, "I'm really just enabling her to live in an inappropriate place, and not really get the care she needs . . . She doesn't understand the risk she is living at." Yet at the same time as she worries about Eleanor's competence to make decisions and her lack understanding of her risks, the case manager still sees her as having ultimate responsibility for her situation: "I am supporting her to the best of my ability based on what she tells me she wants, and will accept, and she is the one who is really master of her destiny."

In this case, the case manager and Eleanor have different ideas of what would help the situation but, I would argue, this is not what explains the dissonance that I think enters the case manager's account at this point. This tension lies not in the case manager's account of her practice, which I read as enacting a logic of care, but in her final statement, that in the end, it is Eleanor who is in control of her destiny. The case manager's practice demonstrates persistence and specificity: staying with Eleanor despite or perhaps because of the difficulties of her life and her personality, trying to figure out what would work best with this person who seems to demand, at the very least, that her particularity be attended to. The case manager tinkers—a little of this, a little of that—but does not try not to fix the situation once and for all, or least not until now. Rather she has tried to improve it. She does not do everything Eleanor wants but tries to support her, to help her to stay safe and reasonably comfortable. In fact, though events have not unfolded smoothly, it seems fair to say that the case manager has been doing what she can, watching out for and trying to respond to problems as they emerge as a result of Eleanor's changing physical and cognitive capabilities (Mol 2008, 79). As well, it also seems likely that it has been the case manager's involvement, particularly the ways that she has built up a loose network of supportive conditions around Eleanor, that has allowed Eleanor to exercise any control at all over events. As Law (1994) might say, she has not treated Eleanor as an actor, able to manage or not manage the conditions of life, but she has acted as though the conditions of Eleanor's life were a network that could be improved in order to better upkeep her existence. As Law writes, "each one of us is an arrangement. That arrangement is more or less fragile. There are ordering processes which keep (or fail to keep) that arrangement on the road" (33). So it is not that Eleanor is the "master of her destiny" but that the case manager's practical activities have contributed to creating the kind of situation in which Eleanor may still make some choices. She is, so to speak, helping to keep her on the road. The case manager, however, does not appear to see this. Rather, she locates control within Eleanor and in so doing makes her responsible for whatever happens next. At this point, practice informed by a logic of care—attentive, variable, flexible—seems to recede, and for me, a certain incoherence enters the case manager's account.

As Mol (2008) observes, the logic of choice is more and more being drawn into practices of health care, and it is not that choice is in itself a bad thing but that the logic of choice, like the logic of care, "carries a whole world with it: a specific mode of organizing action and interaction; of understanding bodies, people and daily lives; of dealing with knowledge and technologies; of distinguishing between good and bad" (7). One of the most concerning features of this world, along with fixing conditions of life as alternatives among which we may choose, are the ways in which the logic of choice positions people primarily as individualized decision makers, instituting expectations that they will rationally manage their lives, including those aspects that may shape their particular vulnerabilities (Ceci and Purkis 2009). It is this that seems incongruent in the case manager's account. Certainly, by drawing on the logic of choice at this moment and centering an ability to make choices within Eleanor, the case manager does set out boundaries of responsibility that may release her from the time-consuming, resource-consuming business of continuing to attend to the difficulties of Eleanor's life, a form of practice that current organizational arrangements do not really seem to support.

Instead, the dominant idea that organizes practice in this setting stresses quite simply that case managers offer alternatives and clients make choices. This is an idea of practice that seems good, not only efficient but protective of clients' agency, choices and autonomy. However it is also a framing of practice that suggests that both case managers and clients are best conceived of as autonomous decisions makers, and one effect of this conceptualization is that practice begins to be seen, as noted above, as a largely rational encounter between 'free agents' working together towards shared goals. This expectation is inscribed and confirmed in other organizational locations. For example, the guiding philosophy of the Long Term Care program affirms the appropriateness of a world ordered by ideals of choice, autonomy and independence: "the underlying principle of the program is the belief that individuals are responsible and wish to care for themselves and their families as long as they are able to do so" (Ministry of Health Services n.d. 5). Case managers are urged to base their practices on values of personal independence, and the promotion of personal and family responsibility.

LOGICS THAT PUSH AND PULL (2)

Though the situation described above is not entirely typical, when I asked case managers to give accounts of their practices, accounts that would shed light on what that practice was like, they invariably offered examples in which the organizational ideal of practice was not particularly helpful. These were not always cases where resources were insufficient, though this did play a role, but cases where clients refused offered and apparently needed services. In these situations, the case managers described clients as exercising their right to make choices and, in some cases, as choosing to live at risk by refusing the services offered. That is, the gap between the sorts of services and support that people were offered and what they might actually need to live their lives was more likely to be explained as an outcome of the client's free choices rather than as representing a failure of care. Yet it seems unlikely that questions of daily life are best settled episodically, in these moments of choosing, once and for all. Rather, the logic and language of 'choice' provides a way out when routinized practice shows itself as unable to address needs or actually respond to people's specific situations; proceduralism is preserved by making events, in the end, a matter of people's choices.

This is not to suggest that practices informed by a logic of choice are inevitably 'bad' but rather that both choice and care arrive with their own good and bad; each kind of practice, as noted previously, brings its own world (Mol 2008, 7). Though Mol's analysis is much more complete, in a nutshell, the logic of choice offers people the possibility of autonomy; without choice, people may be oppressed. Practices informed by a logic of care work towards something different: responsiveness, specificity and making life livable. And in Mol's care-specific terms, "care is bad when people are being neglected" (84). But much of the time, including in home care for older people who are frail, everything arrives together—practices are messy and their logics are not singular. In home care, managerialism, choice and care ebb and flow, each orienting the work differently—a problem for care, however, is that the conditions of practice increasingly limit the logic of care as a defining repertoire for practice. Instead, case managers, possibly in the face of the intensifying bureaucratization, highlight the need to safeguard autonomy, most often understood narrowly as the positive possibility of persons' capacity make 'free' choices about how they will live their lives.

For some case managers, protecting this idea of autonomy becomes central to how they conduct themselves—despite the dissonance that may accompany its enactment. Eva Garden, for example, is an elderly woman, blind and with a variety of health concerns, who has steadfastly refused to leave the dilapidated trailer in which she lives with her daughter, who suffers her own mental health issues. We drive to visit her. The trailer is tiny, dirty, damp, with inadequate plumbing and, to me, appears scarcely habitable, but as her case manager tells me, Eva is very proud to own her own home and has, in the past, refused cleaner and safer accommodation. Yet the conditions in which she lives are such that the home support workers who are contracted to help her with personal care refuse to visit. The case manager responds by tinkering around the edges of the situation. When things get too bad, she arranges a "major cleaning" (Ceci, case manager interview). When sewage starts to back up into the kitchen sink, a situation actually outside her purview, she tracks down a plumber and persuades him to volunteer to fix it. Though she finds the situation in many ways intolerable, she also sees it, in the end, as an outcome of her client's choice: "even if it's not a risk, people make choices. Again, I mean, I guess it's just about our role. And what is our role? . . . Is it really to guide people along a path we want them to take?" She suggests that even more damaging to this woman than living in a decaying trailer would be insisting she be re-housed—that would be "interfering with her freedoms." But knowing she is supporting her client's choices does not resolve her angst about the situation or her anticipation that the situation will worsen: "I'm just waiting for a natural crisis which will be [she] will end up in the hospital." The case manager is keenly aware that failing to respect Eva's 'choices', for example calling in authorities to inspect the property, may 'oppress' her and equally aware that failing to act to improve the situation may result in neglect. So she does what she can but anticipates that it will not be sufficient, that Eva's condition will inevitably deteriorate. This reads like neglect, knowingly allowing deterioration, but what are the options? One thing is clear: while explaining the situation with reference to Eva's free choices does work to set out boundaries of responsibility, it does little to resolve questions of how to work so that Eva's daily life is as good as it can be (Ceci, field notes).

Interestingly, another case manager used almost identical language to account for her practice in a situation in which she attempted to respect a client's expressed desire to remain in her own home despite signs of her deteriorating cognitive status. Helen lived alone and had no family living locally. In this case there was a build-up of signs that "Helen was slipping": she was incontinent at times, missing medications and having trouble letting home support workers into her building, which was on a secure intercom system.[6] The case manager deployed a range of strategies to address these issues. She reorganized Helen's medications so that they would be taken three rather than four times per day and then added an extra 15-minute lunch time visit for a medication reminder. She arranged to have pull-up incontinence pads laid out with Helen's night things with the hope that she would know they were for her to put on. When Helen was incontinent in a chair, she arranged for extra time to have the chair cleaned. And she arranged a routine to assist Helen to remember how to open her front door: "basically she sits in the living room, with a little table with a phone on it, with a note that says 'Press 6 to let someone in'." Eventually Helen can no longer be sustained by this sort of episodic care, workers in and out, visiting regularly although infrequently. She cannot get up from her chair by herself and the case manager concludes "that she really couldn't be on her own." At this point the case manager is able to "patch together hourly blocks of time" so that Helen would not be left alone until she can be "emergency-placed" in a care facility (Ceci, field notes and case manager interview).

There is so much about this situation that seems inadequate in terms of care, and the case manager seems aware of this: "you just go through the dilemma of, is it better to let her have her own way? And that's being client centered with your care. And then you deal with the crisis when it happens? Or when the crisis happens, which is now. . . have we been remiss?" A difficulty for the provision of 'good care' here is that this case manager is solidly positioned in two ways: first, to enact a logic of choice as 'the' way to ensure her care is patient centered, and second, to conceptualize, and limit, her possibilities for action through organizational guidelines that frame interventions in the discourse of hours and minutes of calculable service. Though each may be necessary neither is adequate to the situation. Yet although she wonders if practice in this situation has been inadequate, has been lacking in care, she also observes "you're doing a lot of management by crisis and who's to say that's wrong?" And this seems to me precisely the difficulty. In these situations, in situations where the question is how one is going to be able to live one's life, it is not at all clear what should be done. And it is this—the essential undecidability of how to live—that is unhappily resolved by, is diminished by, reliance on either proceduralism or a logic of choice as grounds for action (Ceci, case manager interview).

WHAT IS GOOD CARE *LIKE*?

To return to the question of what is good care, or rather the question of what good care in home care is *like*, it seems that when practice begins from a place where people are understood as rational, choosing actors, with independence an inherent capacity and normal state as well as both a goal and philosophy, something like 'good care' is less likely to follow. The force of choice as a regulative ideal and proceduralism as the necessary logic of good management crowd out the ways in which home care, as a practice, might actually work to support the constitution of these capabilities—that is, some form of autonomy or independence—for people whose questions concern how to make daily life as livable as possible. Yet there is a strong tendency to assume, in practice arrangements and policy discourses, that people—not just older people but all people—arrive already fully constituted, with service, supports, resources, family, as 'add-ons' to a self-contained and sustaining individualism. This assumption is arguably harder to sustain in the face of frailty, where the nature of sustaining relations and arrangements become in some sense more visible, or at least less invisible. The conditions necessary to live a life are not so easy to overlook. Yet problematically for home care, the inadequacies of sustaining conditions are misread as individualized deficiencies or the cause of frailty. This exchange between a case manager and myself illustrates the naturalness of this frame of reference. She was talking with me about how, after performing her various assessments related to health and activities of daily living, she determines the appropriate level of care[7] to assign to a client:

> *Case manager:* One of the things I do is say, what would this person be like if there were no supports in place at all? So how do they stand, completely naked of any other resources? That helps me a lot, to make that decision.
> *C. Ceci:* Do you mean non-professional resources?
> *Case manager:* Or professional resources, everything, like informal, formal, volunteers, family, private pay. . . If they didn't have any of that, what would it look like?
> *(Ceci, case manager interview)*

In some respects this seems a promising, even sensible, starting point for a case management practice oriented to providing supportive assistance to older people. Except does anyone exist without resources? Or rather, can anyone sustain existence without connection to a diverse assortment of socio-material structures and supports (Moser 2006)? How is it helpful to metaphorically strip the person of all attachments and to consider this as in some sense a 'natural' state, or a state that reveals some essential truth about the person? The case manager's framing suggests that it is not only possible but makes sense to grasp the person as separate and separable from her world, and also that it is the inability to stand naked without resources, a deficiency of the person, that will call for her intervention. My difficulty here is not that her interventions will take the form of strategies intended to supplement perceived gaps in a client's support network, but that these actions are understood as compensation for the *client's* lack or loss. Her work takes the form of normalizing the situation, enacting the assumption that *normally*, people are able to stand naked, are responsible for themselves (Moser 2005). And it is this assumption and all that follows from it, that I think can be called into question. To return to Law's words, "each one of us is an arrangement. That arrangement is more or less fragile. There are ordering processes which keep (or fail to keep) that arrangement on the road" (1994, 33).

NOTES

1. Findings from the research referred to in this paper have been reported elsewhere—see Ceci 2006a, 2006b, 2008; Ceci and Purkis 2009, 2010 for study details. In this chapter, the intent is to rethink these analyses in light of new thinking and this new question.
2. See also Joanna Latimer, this volume.
3. Case managers in the jurisdiction in which this study was conducted are overwhelming women. Most have nursing degrees (BN or MN), although some positions are filled by social workers. The preponderance of nurses does suggest that in some respects this is still seen as a 'health' role.
4. The field study was focused on observations of, and conversations about, the events and activities of case management practice, including home visits with new clients, reassessments of long-time clients, connecting with family, both locally and at a distance, as well as coordinating the work of other involved health workers. Alongside case managers, I observed unit meetings, program meetings, and hospital and community rounds. Other data collection activities were interviews with managers of various aspects of the Home and Community Care programs and the analysis of the text-based information that influences the work: forms, memos, procedure manuals, the regional health plan and so on. Analysis of data was ongoing and iterative and undertaken in light of current writings in home care as well as critical health, social and philosophical theory more generally.
5. Based on case managers' assessments (excepting the financial ones), clients are categorized or assigned one of five possible care levels: personal care (PC), intermediate care (IC 1–3), extended care (EC). Care levels are linked with assessed needs and come with pre-authorized maximum amounts and types of services to meet those needs.
6. People at the front entrance would telephone up to her apartment and she would have to press a code to release the front door lock.
7. See note 5.

REFERENCES

Andrews, Gavin. 2003. Locating a geography of nursing: space, place and the progress of geographical thought. *Nursing Philosophy* 4: 231–248.

Angus, Jan, Pia Kontos, Isabel Dyck, Patricia McKeever and Blake Poland. 2005. The personal significance of home: habitus and the experience of receiving long-term home care. *Sociology of Health and Illness* 27(2): 161–187.

Aronson, Jane and Sheila Neysmith. 2006. Obscuring the costs of home care: restructuring at work. *Work, Employment and Society* 20: 27–45.

Baranek Patricia M., Raisa B. Deber and A. Paul Williams. 2004. *Almost home: Reforming home and community care in Ontario*. Toronto: University of Toronto Press.

Bauman, Zygmunt. 2002. The fate of humanity in a post-Trinitarian world. *Journal of Human Rights* 1(3): 283–303.

Burchall, Graham, Colin Gordon and Peter Miller. 1991. Preface. In *The Foucault effect: Studies in governmentality*, edited by Graham Burchell, Colin Gordon and Peter Miller, ix–x. Chicago: University of Chicago Press.

Ceci, Christine. 2006a. Impoverishment of practice: analysis of effects of economic discourses in home care case management. *Canadian Journal of Nursing Leadership* 19(1): 56–68.

——— 2006b. "What she says she needs doesn't make a lot of sense": practices of seeing in home care case management. *Nursing Philosophy* 7: 90–99.

——— 2008. Increasingly distant from life: problem setting in the organization of home care. *Nursing Philosophy* 9: 19–31.

Ceci, Christine, and Mary Ellen Purkis. 2009. Bridging gaps in risk discourse: home care case management and client choices. *Sociology of Health and Illness* 31(2): 201–214.

——— 2010. Implications of an epistemological vision: Knowing what to do in home care. In *Rebirth of the clinic: Places and agents in contemporary health care*, edited by Cindy Patton, 17–38. Minneapolis: University of Minnesota Press.

——— 2011. Means without ends: Justifying supportive home care for frail older people in Canada, 1990–2010. *Sociology of Health and Illness* DOI: 10.111/j.1467-9566.2011.01344x.

Coyte, Peter and Patricia McKeever. 2001. Home care in Canada: passing the buck. *Canadian Journal of Nursing Research* 33(2): 11–25.

Duncan Susan and Linda Reutter. 2006. A critical policy analysis of an emerging agenda for home care in one Canadian province. *Health and Social Care in the Community* 14(3): 242–253.

Flood, Colleen. 1999. *Unpacking the shift to home care*. Halifax, NS: Maritime Centre of Excellence for Women's Health.

Foucault, Michel. 1989. Problematics. In *Foucault live: Collected interviews, 1961–1984*, edited by Sylvere Lotringer, translated by Lysa Hochroth and John Johnson, 416–422. New York: Semiotext(e).

——— 1991. Questions of method. In *The Foucault effect: Studies in governmentality*, edited by Graham Burchell, Colin Gordon and Peter Miller, 73–86. Chicago: University of Chicago Press.

Gregor, Fran. 1997. From women to women: nurses, informal caregivers and the gender dimension of health care reform in Canada. *Health and Social Care in the Community* 5(1): 30–36.

Hollander, Marcus. 2003. *Unfinished business: The case for chronic home care services, a policy paper*. Victoria: Hollander Analytical Services.

Hollander, Marcus and Nina Chappell. 2002. *Final report of the National Evaluation of the Cost-effectiveness of Home Care, A report prepared for the Health Transition Fund, Health Canada*. Victoria: National Evaluation of the Cost–Effectiveness of Home Care.

Hollander, Marcus and Michael Prince. 2007. Organizing healthcare delivery systems for persons with ongoing care needs and their families: a best practices framework. Healthcare Quarterly 11(1): 42–52.

Law, John. 1994. *Organizing modernity*. Oxford: Blackwell.

Ministry of Health Services. n.d. *Home and community care policy manual: School of case management*. Victoria, BC: Author.

Mol, Annemarie. 2008. *The logic of care: Health and the problem of patient choice*. London: Routledge.

Moser, Ingunn. 2005. On becoming disabled and articulating alternatives: the multiple modes of ordering disability and their interferences. *Cultural Studies* 19(6): 667–700.

——— 2006. Sociotechnical practices and differences: on the interferences between disability, gender, and class. *Science, Technology & Human Values* 31(5): 537–564.

———— 2010. Perhaps tears should not be counted but wiped away: On quality and improvement in dementia care. In *Care in Practice: On tinkering in clinics, homes and farms*, edited by Annemarie Mol, Ingunn Moser and Jeanette Pols, 277ñ300. Bielefeld: Transcript Verlag

Pringle, Dorothy. 2006. Home care: we want more. *Canadian Journal of Nursing Leadership* 19: 1.

Purkis, Mary Ellen. 2001. Managing home nursing care: visibility, accountability and exclusion. *Nursing Inquiry* 8(3): 141–150.

Purkis, Mary Ellen, Christine Ceci and Kristin Björnsdottir. 2008. Patching up the holes: analysing the work of home care. *Canadian Journal of Public Health* 99(S2): S27–S32.

Rozanova, Julia, Herbert C. Northcott and Susan McDaniel. 2006. Seniors and portrayals of intra-generational and inter-generational inequality in the *Globe and Mail*. *Canadian Journal on Ageing* 25(4): 373–386.

Romanow, Roy. 2002. *Discussion paper: Homecare in Canada*. Ottawa: Commission of the Furture of Health Care in Canada and Canadian Health Services Research Foundation.

Struhkamp, Rita, Annemare Mol and Tsjalling Swierstra. 2008. Dealing with in/dependence: doctoring in Physical Rehabilitation practice. *Science, Technology & Human Values* 34: 55–76.

Twigg, Julia. 2006. *The body in health and social care*. New York: Palgrave Macmillan.

5   Bringing It All Back Home

The (Re)Domestication and (De)Medicalization of Care in the UK

Davina Allen

For 60 years in modern healthcare systems the hospital has been the preferred site of care. However care is currently undergoing a process of (re) domestication and (de)medicalization. Owing to a combination of economic, demographic and ideological factors, 'home care' has gradually come to be regarded as the gold standard for the organization of care in both institutional and domiciliary contexts. While home care policies serve a range of professional and political agenda, they contain unacknowledged contradictions and strains for the cared-for, families and waged carers. In this paper I draw on two ethnographic studies of caring work undertaken in the United Kingdom (UK) over the last decade (Allen 2000a, 2000b, 2002a, 2002b) and scholarship on 'home-care' in the context of dying (Exley and Allen 2007) to examine some effects of these trends on the caring division of labor, our understanding of social and health care and the relationship between caring about someone and caring for them.

Background

Historically, most health care was provided in the home by members of the household or, for the wealthier middle classes, by domestic servants. With developments in medicine, the hospital increasingly came to be regarded as the preferred site of care and, in the UK for the best part of a century, care has been provided in institutional settings. Reflecting these broader trends, the licence and mandate of the nursing professions has been constructed around claims about a distinctive expertise in care-giving.

Like many modern healthcare systems, the UK caring division of labor is currently undergoing a process of (re)domestication and (de)medicalization, producing shifts in the contexts of care and a redistribution of caring functions away from nurses to family members and/or significant others and 'social' care providers. Healthcare is increasingly underpinned by the assumption that in all but the most acute cases, home is the preferred site of care; that families should care for dependent relatives and that certain kinds of care may be designated as a 'social' rather than a 'health' need.

The privileging of home care as a model for the social organization of caring work is based on several implicit assumptions about 'home' as a social space, the nature of the relationships therein and their implications for the organization of caregiving. Home care is assumed to be founded on loving relationships and the social obligations that arise from ties of marriage and kinship. Caring about someone (having caring feelings) is assumed to be a foundation for caring for them (carrying out caring work). Home is taken to be a place in which individuals are relaxed and at their ease, where privacy can be maintained and choice and agency assured. This characterization of home care can be contrasted to institutional care in which caring work is based on an economic contract. In this context it is the needs of the organization that determine the arrangements for care. Here, batch-living, people processing, and time scheduling objectify the patient and militate against privacy, choice and control.

In the UK the idea of home care emerged in the context of the 1959 Mental Health Act and was very quickly extended to all client groups. An initial emphasis on care *in* the community shifted during the 1970s to an emphasis on care *by* the community (Finch 1990). These policy trends were the result of a coalescence of several different pressures: an ageing population, public expenditure contraction and a marriage of left-wing critiques of institutional care with right-wing policies emphasizing self-help and the family. In the intervening period, home care policies have been reinforced by consumerist ideologies that have stressed greater public involvement and by a rolling back of the state that has redrawn the boundaries between 'health' and 'social' care. These trends have gained momentum despite recognition that traditional models of family support are not available to all, owing to geographic mobility, the changing role of women and the number of one-parent families and people living alone.

The Data

This paper draws on ethnographic data generated in two previously published studies of caring work. Study 1 examined interprofessional and interagency working in the care of adults who had suffered a first acute stroke (Allen et al. 2000; Allen, Griffiths and Lyne 2004a, 2004b). The research was carried out in two sites and four case studies were undertaken in each. The 'case' comprised the client and their network of care as they progressed from acute hospital to home or community care. Data were generated over six months through interviews with health and social service providers, observations and audio-recordings of key meetings. Case notes and additional documentation were also sources of data. Fieldwork was undertaken by a research assistant on each site. Data generation, coding and analysis were undertaken concurrently and involved all members of the research team.

Study 2 focused on how nurses, patients and families negotiated care in the acute context (Allen 2000a, 2000b, 2002a, 2002b). Although not directly concerned with home care, the research produced insights into the implications of the changing role of family carers for the social organization of care work. The study was undertaken on a surgical and a medical ward in a large UK teaching hospital. Data comprise fieldnotes generated as a participant observer, audio-recorded interviews with nurses and health-care assistants and interviews with patients and their carers recorded contemporaneously in a field diary.

Signed consent was obtained from all patients, family and friends directly participating in each study. Ethical approvals were granted by the relevant Research Ethics Committee. All participants are referred to by pseudonyms.

Both studies were informed by sociological theories of the division of labor in which care was defined as work, irrespective of the identity of the caregiver or the nature of the relationship on which caregiving was predicated. The primary focus was the negotiation of care work in every-day practice with data generation designed to address the following broad questions: what kinds of work does the provision of health and social care entail? Who does that work and what is the knowledge that underpins it? How is the work negotiated between those involved? What effect does context have on all of the above? Findings from both studies have been reported elsewhere (Allen 2000a, 2000b, 2002a, 2002b; Allen, Griffiths and Lyne 2004a, 2004b).

For the purposes of this chapter, I want to draw on these microlevel observations, to ask some macro-level questions in order to progress theory and practice in this field. In doing so, I will be building on ideas expressed in a related body of scholarship on the caring division of labor in general (Allen 2001, 2004, 2007; Dingwall and Allen 2001) and the extension of this thinking to care of the dying in particular (Exley and Allen 2007). The latter work arose out of collaborative scholarship which brought together complementary interests in care of the dying (Exley) and the caring division of labour (Allen) to revisit interviews generated in a series of studies on experiences of home care at the end of life (Exley 1999; Exley and Letherby 2001; Exley et al. 2005; Exley and Tyrer 2005; McKinley et al. 2004).

HOME CARE POLICIES: IMPLICATIONS FOR 'CARE'

Home care policies present fundamental challenges to the existing caring division of labor, calling into question understanding of what it means to care in modern society. I am going to critically examine several issues that arise from these trends for those cared for, families and waged carers.

Negotiating Caring Expertise

The nursing professions have evolved and developed in parallel with the rise of the modern hospital, and nursing jurisdiction has been pushed and pulled in different directions.

One key development has been a more active engagement with, and recognition of, the contribution of family carers. Drawing on Harvath et al. (1994), Nolan, Grant and Keady (1996) suggest that high quality care emerges from the skillful blending of the local knowledge of family caregivers with the generic knowledge of formal carers. However, in practice this blending of 'lay' and 'professional' knowledge can be difficult to effect.

In Study 2 I identified that family members who had previously been caring for their relative prior to their admission to hospital (referred to as 'expert carers') presented particular challenges for ward staff (Allen 2000b). Expert family caregivers not only have a knowledge of the cared-for person's needs derived from their relationship and experience of their response to illness, they also develop their own understanding of how to care for their loved one and this can conflict with the views of healthcare providers. In a previously published paper, I described the case of Mrs. Durham and her efforts to influence the care of her husband, John. Mrs. Durham had been caring for John at home after he had suffered a stroke. He had difficulty swallowing and this had resulted in food and drink entering his lungs, causing pneumonia. During his hospitalization health providers decided John required an artificial feeding tube. Mrs. Durham strongly resisted this idea, despite the pressure being applied by the multidisciplinary team:

> The other day there was a whole group of them there—the speech therapist, physio, a couple of nurses and some others that I didn't know—and they'd come to try and persuade me to let him have the PEG (artificial feeding tube). They seemed to want me to make a decision right away and I didn't want to so I said, "You can all go away and I will think about it." A little later a nurse came back on the same deposition. In the end I went home and I telephoned my GP (General Practitioner), who I know and trust, and he explained it all to me and why he felt I should let the experts guide me. (Fieldnotes)

Eventually it was agreed that an artificial feeding tube would not be passed, but that John should only receive thickened fluids and pureed food to minimize the risk of further respiratory complications. The speech and language therapist left guidance as to how he should be fed, but Mrs. Durham devised her own instructions.

Mrs. Durham has left instructions for feeding John for a meal on Monday evening. She begins by saying how much she thinks John is likely to want to eat.

Mrs. Durham: I could have written more but I didn't think anyone would read it.

DA: The speech and language therapist left some explicit instructions in the notes but I guess it would be useful to have them here for people to refer to.

Mrs. Durham: But even the speech and language therapist wasn't feeding him properly. She was going too fast. She was giving him too much. Even three-quarters of a teaspoon is too much. She was putting it into the middle of his mouth but it's better to put it on the right side because the muscles are better on the right. And he needs to be told to swallow each time. (Fieldnotes)

Mrs. Durham's challenges to medical expertise became a source of increasing tension and John was eventually moved to another ward on the grounds that he had a fecal infection and should be nursed in a single room. However, given that he was never actually nursed in isolation (the nurses on the second ward said it was unnecessary) and no attempt was made to move another patient who had the same infection, it seems reasonable to infer that John was moved not exclusively for clinical reasons.

Staff Nurse: Have you seen Mrs. Durham lately?

DA: Are they still in?

Staff Nurse (rolls her eyes): I don't know. The last I heard he was on Poppy Ward. I thought he'd come back when his clostridium was resolved.

DA: He was out on the ward before it was resolved.

Staff Nurse: Oh well it was an excuse to get him into a cubicle. You need to share people like that, don't you? (Fieldnotes)

It is not my intention to demonize the health providers in this case. They were sympathetic to Mrs. Durham's perspective, but the continuing disagreements about John's care exhausted their time and energy. What is of significance, however, is that these tensions around expertise inhibited any deeper communication about his interests. Having observed the situation from both sides over several days, I spent time talking to John's daughter when she visited her father one weekend. She referred to herself as having entered a "battleground" and described the emotional labor she had expended supporting her mother "in hysterics" on the telephone every evening. Our conversation was informative and added a previously unacknowledged insight into this very difficult situation.

And now his swallowing has gone—that's really awful. She said that if he can't eat or drink wine then what quality of life has he got then? She's also a bit squeamish and doesn't fancy the tube into the stomach. (Fieldnotes)

Thus it would seem that Mrs. Durham's resistance to the feeding tube reflected a desire to preserve the only thing of value she perceived her husband had left: eating and drinking. Furthermore, owing to her "squeamishness," she may also have feared that if the feeding tube was passed she would be unable to continue to care for him at home. It is clear that in John's case, healthcare professionals' recommendations were based on a biomedical understanding of John's individual 'need', whereas Mrs. Durham's resistance was filtered through broader social concerns about sustaining a normal life for *herself and* her husband. However, because the situation was framed as a dispute over expertise, the question of whether John should continue feeding normally in full recognition of the risks was never broached.

This example highlights several implications for the caring division of labor raised by home care policies. First, these trends are producing a redistribution of caring expertise. An important consequence of encouraging family caregiving is a narrowing of the gap in knowledge between professional and lay carers and a transfer of power and control. The occupational socialization of nursing emphasizes engagement with subjectivities and "knowing the patient" (Armstrong 1983; May 1992). Yet when both nurses and family carers claim to know the patient, who is best placed to assess an individual's interest? Second, these tensions are exacerbated because health professionals and family carers come to know the patient and constitute need within different interpretative frames. In this example, nurses and healthcare providers defined need from within a narrow biomedical perspective, where the primary concern was avoiding pneumonia. Mrs. Durham understood need from within a social perspective in which the primary concern was normalization. Third, these negotiations do not take place in a vacuum but are shaped by the social relations in which caregiving is embedded and the wider priorities and concerns of those involved (Allen, Griffiths, and Lyne 2004b). In this case, Mrs. Durham's understanding of need was shaped by her affective relationship with her husband and her desire for him to remain at home. Ward staff actions were shaped by biomedical concerns and wider work pressures. Given these considerations, we can see that developing satisfactory relationships between family and professional carers is infinitely more complex than blending local and global caring expertise. Such expertise and understanding of 'need' is constituted within quite different interpretative frames and colored in important ways by the different concerns of healthcare providers and family members.

Caring For and Caring About: Bodies and Identity

Home care policies take social relationships as the prerequisite for family care rather than skills and knowledge. However, the 'rosy' images that surround the idea of family caregiving mask the physical, economic and emotional costs that such activity can entail (Henwood 1990 cited by Tarraborreli 1994). Since the middle ages modern societies have been involved in a civilising process in which we have come to see our bodies as encasing ourselves. Elias (1983) has argued that from the 1500s to 1900s an "invisible wall of affects" arose between bodies, with individuals being embarrassed or uncomfortable with the bodily functions of others as well as having their own bodily functions exposed. Contemporary conceptions of home care fail to recognize that a whole range of bodily and biological processes have become individualized and privatized, and community knowledge about bodies and bodily care has been increasingly appropriated by professional carers. Thus, whilst providing intimate bodily care is an acceptable part of familial adult-child relations, in modern western societies it is not an expectation of close adult relationships. With the rise of the modern hospital, body work has been under the control of nurses and has become largely hidden from view. Despite the growing corpus of nursing scholarship, little attention has been paid to nurses' work with bodies and nurses do not foreground this work in their public professional claims, emphasizing instead their technical and interpersonal caring expertise. One consequence of this is that knowledge about how bodies behave when they are malfunctioning or in decline has become lost from the community, and this can create very real challenges for family members faced with the expectation to care for dependent relatives.

Evidence of such tensions can be found in a previously published paper on home care policies in the context of dying (Exley and Allen 2007). Interviews with people who were dying revealed that many had concerns about whether they would become dependent on caregivers for bodily care and whether family members were able to undertake this role.

> I worry about what's coming next for me. What physical symptoms will I get next? Wonder whether they'll be, whether I'll be reliant on him [her husband] for my personal things you know. I'm looking after myself at the moment, but there will be a time when I can't do that sort of thing for myself, I don't like to talk about that. Because I think it worries him that he might not be able to cope with that. (Interview—Liz)

Here Liz expresses her concerns that she will become dependent on her husband for her "personal things" and that he might not be able to cope with this care need. Interestingly, however, this is not an issue they have discussed explicitly. The ideal of home care is based on the strength of social ties as the basis for caring relationships; however, emotional intimacy can actually make the demands of bodily care more difficult and challenge the very relationship on which care-giving is founded. In the context of nursing, Lawler (1991) has questioned whether emotional intimacy is an appropriate basis for body work. She argues that, given the taboos that mark these social boundaries, body care is made more manageable by the adoption of a detached, emotionally remote stance. Social relationships can be changed and challenged by body work and intimately caring for a spouse can impact negatively on sexual relationships (Parker 1993) as the case of Jane and her husband illustrates.

> Jane is a woman in her early 40s. Her husband David died of a brain tumour. Throughout his illness Jane, her father and some friends cared for David at home. They had little input from formal health-care services. Although caring for David in the latter stages of his illness was demanding it was something Jane felt she wanted to do. Jane and David had an 11-year-old daughter, and having her dying father at home had an impact on her. As David's physical condition deteriorated Jane found it increasingly difficult to cope. Towards the end of his life David became doubly incontinent. She found changing his catheter tube difficult and physically and emotionally uncomfortable for both of them and this job was often left to male friends or Jane's father. One night Jane and her daughter had to move David from his bed to the bath to clean him up after he had soiled himself. She spoke about how difficult it was to ask her daughter to help move her father in 'that state', but that she was unable to move him on her own. Having managed to get David into the bath they were unable to move him again, and he spent the remainder of that night in the bath, naked, covered with a duvet, which Jane found distressing. For Jane providing this personal intimate care was extremely difficult, she felt that doing this somehow destroyed the previous sexually intimate relationship she had had with her husband. Shortly after the episode described David was admitted to a private hospital (unusually) to die. Jane spoke about his admission with palpable relief. She talked about how she felt she had got her husband back in those last few weeks of life. Jane and their daughter were able to go to the hospital, sit in David's private room, take in special picnics and their favourite wine. His personal care was no longer her responsibility and, albeit in an alien environment, their identities as partners and parents were re-established before David's death. (Fieldnotes)

As this example demonstrates, home care privileges caring relationships without acknowledging the interaction of pre-existing social ties with the actual work of caring. The same social identities that provided the initial foundation for their caring relationships were also the cause of their distress. These issues may arguably be magnified in the context of social expectations that children care for their frail elder parents. Much of the feminist-inspired analysis of caring has downplayed its affective components in order to highlight its status as unpaid work, rather than a labor of love. However, these data suggests that any conceptualization of home care practice has to bring these affective relationships into view.

Who Cares? Obligation and Choice

There is an assumption in social policy that informal care comes first and that outside agencies need only step in if this is unavailable (Twigg and Atkin 1994). Because home care policies assume that caring about someone should be the foundation for caring for them, it is very difficult for families to assert their own needs without fear of social censure. A willingness to care for someone is taken as an indicator of the moral status of a relationship. Thus, whilst social ties are taken to be the basis for home care, these may be called into question if, for whatever reason, families are unable or do not wish to care for their relative at home. The needs of the cared-for and their families are not necessarily synonymous. Finding a workable package which bridges both parties' needs can be extremely difficult and the constraints within which health and social service providers operate can exert pressures on families to accept arrangements which may not be in their long-term interests. The case of Edward in Study 1 highlights these inter-related dilemmas (Allen, Griffiths, and Lyne 2004b).

Edward was admitted to hospital following a left frontal lobe infarction resulting in a right-sided paralysis and difficulties in processing and formulating language. He was married with one son and his wife was pregnant with twins. Edward was in hospital for eight months, during which time his coordination improved, but he was left with profound communication difficulties. A variety of discharge packages were explored and eventually he was placed in a residential home, where he settled well. However, planning for Edward's discharge highlighted a conflict between his desire to return home and the needs of his wife (Rhonda), who felt unable to cope. This produced a division within the health and social care team. On one side were Edward and the speech and language therapist, who wanted a home discharge. On the other were Rhonda and the social worker, who claimed that a home discharge was unsustainable. At the multidisciplinary meetings convened to discuss Edward's continuing care, Rhonda (RM) was pressured by the speech and language therapist (SALT) to take him home.

> *SALT to RM:* It's the communication that bothers you most?
>
> *RM:* Mmm. Yeah, because it's no, you can't have a (. . .) he can't come up and tell me. You know? "I want this" or you know? [. . .] He couldn't tell me "I'm tired" or "I've got a pain here." He can't describe things to me.
>
> *SALT:* What about then if you asked him questions based on what you think it might be?
>
> *RM:* Yeah, but I'm there forever aren't I? (Gives example)
>
> [. . .]

> SALT: So, you couldn't live with that sort of pressure?
> RM: (.) See, I don't know. I don't know, like I can't say what he would
>   be like at home? (Case conference—audio-recording).

What is interesting about this exchange is the way in which the SALT locates responsibility for the difficulties with the discharge arrangements with Rhonda: it is her inability to cope with the pressure that is putting a home placement in jeopardy. The discussion then moves on to focus on community support. The social worker depicts a rather starker image of the reality of a home discharge than that portrayed by the SALT.

> Social Worker: I think you've got to be aware that if we are going with
>   the home situation, the responsibility is going to be leveled
>   on your shoulders for most of the time [. . .]. So you've got
>   to know what you're taking on and, you know, what the
>   situation is. [. . .] It is a permanent responsibility to know
>   where we're going with that. And I think it is necessary for
>   us to work with that because, you know, for something to
>   last, or to be OK for a couple of months, isn't any good.
>   Because we're not talking about a couple of months.
> SALT: Well if that's the case, Rhonda, basically you're saying that you
>   can't have him home. I'm not trying to put words into your
>   mouth but we have to be clear about what the options are.
>   (Case conference—audio-recording)

These disagreements led to service providers questioning Rhonda's moral integrity. In one multidisciplinary meeting the team expressed suspicion that she was trying to use Edward's condition to assist an application for re-housing even though it had been agreed that he was not returning home.

> Occupational therapist: His wife rang our main department this
>   week. She wanted a copy of my home visit report, regarding
>   housing. And she's seen me since but hasn't acknowledged
>   this, so it's all a bit peculiar. Whether she's trying to go
>   ahead with the housing situation regardless of where's he's
>   going. I'm not sure.
>   [. . .]
> Staff Nurse: I think she is still using his case as the reason to get re-
>   housed. (Multidisciplinary team meeting—audio-recording)

We were unable to establish the veracity of these claims. For current purposes, however, what is of significance is how Rhonda is positioned as not prioritizing Edward's interests. Rhonda realized that this decision had alienated her from certain of the healthcare providers and she formed an alliance with the social worker, who was more sympathetic to her situation.

> *Social Worker:* Rhonda is aware that she's become the villain of the piece.
> *SALT:* What, on the unit?
> *Social Worker:* Yes, she's not stupid. She's confided in me about having him back. It would be the easiest thing in the world for her to have him back, to go along with everything and pretend there's no problem. But she's being very wise. (Fieldnotes)

This formulation of Rhonda's behavior by the social worker—that she is being very wise—contrasts vividly with that of the hospital-based team, who called into question her moral integrity. In some respects, Rhonda was fortunate in finding an ally in the social worker. She also had insider knowledge of the operation of social care provision as a result of her job. Not all families are in the same position and, in the face of pressure from service providers, may accept arrangements because of their perceived social obligations to the detriment of their own wellbeing and that of their relative. There needs to be a greater sensitivity to the moral dilemmas families face and ensure they are given permission to reject home care if it is inappropriate. Some people may want to be cared for at home and have carers who are willing and able to do it, but others may not.

Redefining 'Health' Care and 'Social' Care— Implications for Equality, Equity and Quality

A further consequence of home care policies has been a reconstruction of care needs in terms of 'health' and 'social' provision. In the UK, health care is free as part of the National Health Service (NHS), whereas social care is provided by local authorities and is means-tested. For those individuals who need additional support to remain in their home and/or who cannot rely on family caregivers, this (de)medicalization of care has important implications for equality, equity and quality. In Study 1, in which we examined preparation for discharge in the case of eight adults who had suffered a first acute stroke, those families with access to private resources had greater choice than those dependent on social services provision. To illustrate this point, I am going to take the contrasting cases of Brian and Rosa, previously reported in full in Allen, Griffiths and Lyne (2004a).

An important background factor in understanding these cases is the pressures on bed occupancy in the acute sector and the operation of waiting lists in social services departments in the community. Bed utilization in the acute sector is a key organizational concern, length of stay is carefully monitored and dedicated posts have been implemented specifically to expedite hospital discharge processes. Local councils manage their social care budgets in different ways and use different formulae to assess eligibility. In both cases in this study, in order to manage their fixed budget, the social services departments allocated only a proportion of their funds monthly, and this was managed by a panel that met fortnightly. In the following two cases, we can see how these combined pressures had a differential impact on the service's ability to accommodate the needs of families, and how, in turn, this also shaped relationships between acute sector staff and service users.

Rosa was an 83-year-old widow who had suffered a stroke. She had a supportive family who assisted with cooking, shopping, laundry and cleaning. Initially Rosa made a good recovery and plans were made for her to be discharged to her daughter's home, with support of family and social services funded home care. However, whilst in hospital Rosa suffered another stroke which rendered her incontinent and wheelchair bound. In the light of Rosa's changed needs it was suggested that a nursing home would be a more appropriate discharge destination. In cases where individual needs are complex, nursing home placements are easier for service providers to organize than a home discharge, and given the pressure on acute beds, there is a strain towards this option in order to expedite the discharge process. Rosa was considered to have 'social' rather than 'health' care needs and thus would be expected to contribute to the costs of nursing home care. In the following extract we can see how, in subtle ways, the family is directed towards service provider's preferred option.

> *Son-in-Law:* I am quite happy to support Jayne [Rosa's daughter] in any way I can. I know, like when my mother was ill if somebody had said nursing home, I wouldn't do it. [. . .]
>
> *Social Worker:* You need to go and look at some homes. You are also going to need to talk to the nursing and medical staff here about physically what they do. [. . .] Because you are coming in after work, you need to know literally what, physically, what a day is going to mean for you. [. . .] Can you cope with it? Can you cope with the distress of when you need to move her and she is crying out in pain when there is no way of moving her without pain. (Audio-recorded meeting)

Despite the subtle pressures exerted on them to agree to a nursing home placement, the family insisted they wished to take Rosa home. Given the pressures on acute beds and the time required to organize a complex package of home care, preparation for discharge begins at the earliest opportunity. However, because in this case it was assumed that the family would accept the recommendation for a nursing home discharge, no arrangements had been set in motion. In order to support a home-placement, social services carers were required, along with several items of equipment: bed, cot-sides, a hoist and a commode. Service providers expressed doubt as to whether these arrangements would work and predicted that within a few days Rosa's family would realize that they were unable to cope. A home discharge was eventually arranged, however, and contrary to these pessimistic predictions, Rosa continued to progress and was eventually well enough to attend a local day center once a week. In a striking parallel with the case of Edward, the family's resistance to healthcare professionals' preferred plan for a nursing home placement resulted in strained relations between the family and acute sector staff, who called into question their moral integrity. The family was portrayed as driven by financial motivations rather than by Rosa's interests and their difficulty in reaching a decision was read as a stalling tactic in order to allow them to accommodate a holiday.

> *Health visitor:* The relatives (laughing) they're all keeping an eye on how much money there is available [. . .]
> *GP:* Yeah of course they are.
> *Physiotherapist:* They're well on the ball, they're in front of us, they know *exactly* how much it is going to cost. (Fieldnotes)

> *Ward manager:* The family are going to America.
> *GP:* The daughter who is looking after her is going to America?
> *Occupational Therapist:* They've strung this out really, they knew the equipment was going to take a long time to get.
> *Consultant:* If it's going to take a while she can, she should go into a nursing home until it's ready.
> *Occupational Therapist:* Yes, what about that! (Fieldnotes)

Rosa's case can be contrasted with that of Brian. Brian was 87 when he suffered a right-sided stroke. He lived in a converted barn in the grounds of his son's home. Following his stroke, Brian had extensive nursing needs and would ordinarily have been admitted to a nursing home funded by the local health authority. However, his son wished for him to return home and had the financial means to support him. Brian required a complex package of care that necessitated close collaboration between the family, a private social care agency and the community nursing team. As these arrangements took shape, Brian's care needs were reconstructed in order that they could be accommodated within the jurisdictional boundaries of health and social care providers. This entailed a subtle process in which it was necessary for staff to derive solutions in order to overcome the mismatch between Brian's predominantly health needs and the restricted roles of the social care workers who would be providing most of his on-going care. For example, at the time of the study, home care workers were not permitted to administer prescribed substances. Therefore, in order for them to be able to give Brian the thickened drinks he required, these had to be purchased by the family rather than prescribed by the doctor. This is an option that would not be available to those with more limited economic means. Additionally, as a result of the changed definition of nursing and social care, attending to personal hygiene needs was no longer a health responsibility. However, it was not possible for the home carer to attend to Brian's hygiene needs single-handedly, so in order for the package to work, both community nurses and the home care manager had to be flexible in their local application of formal policies.

> *District nurse team leader:* At the meeting it was agreed that the [private care] agency would be responsible for his hygiene [...] the feeding, the food and everything, and we are responsible for his PEG tube, but they are responsible for the food he eats orally, hum, but they were having problems—some of the carers—with washing and dressing him in the morning, because he's so stiff at times, I mean, I am being quite flexible actually, because I could have said "No, Arthur, you will have to pay for someone else to come in." But as far as I am concerned he is paying out enough money as it is for care to keep his dad at home. We are going there anyway, and I can put his stiffness and his awkwardness, not in himself, in his body down to his medical condition, so I feel that nursing will help. (Interview)

The team's preparedness to negotiate in order to find a suitable care package in Brian's case contrasts with the social worker's emotionally weighted attempt to persuade Rosa's family to accept the preferred option advanced by the professional care team. Brian met the 'continuing care criteria,' which meant that he qualified for health authority funding, and as a consequence, the team were unlikely to incur delays waiting to access funding or equipment through social services. Second, Brian's family had access to considerable private finance to help support the social component of his care and had good quality accommodation that enabled care at home without modification. Finally, and perhaps more significantly, Brian's relatives had the necessary social capital to negotiate the system:

> *Private home care services manager:* He is a very clever gentleman [...] The first thing he did at that meeting was to say several times that he is very ignorant about this, but you can be sure he's not half as ignorant as he was pretending to be [...] he disarmed everybody. Everybody was very helpful, trying to do the best they could for him because he was so nice and grateful and said so many times how well everybody was doing [...] Everybody did everything and he got exactly what he wanted out of that meeting[....] He has got the extra care in the morning and evening [...] without paying for it. He got it. And he manipulated that meeting

totally without anybody suspecting really that he was doing it. (Interview)

As the contrasting cases of Rosa and Brian illustrate, one of the consequences of the changing boundary between definitions of health and social care is significant inequities of service provision and, in the context of the operation of waiting lists for social care services, the development of tensions between the desire of acute sector staff to effect a timely discharge and the needs of families to consider carefully the arrangements which best meet their needs. When accessing funding is not problematic, health and social services staff members were able to collaborate effectively to negotiate integrated services tailored to individual need and devise innovative solutions to circumvent some of the inflexibilities of the system. In instances where families were dependent on social services provision, accommodating need was more difficult, and faced with pressures on acute sector beds, health and social care providers were drawn into enforcing particular solutions in the interests of expediency. This study was undertaken in the UK in the late 1990s, since this time, in the face of growing financial pressures, local councils are increasingly restricting social care to those with the most severe needs. This has left thousands of people without support and forced to pay for private help, move into expensive nursing home care or rely on loved ones to act as unpaid carers.

CONCLUSIONS

In this chapter I have assembled selected findings from a body of scholarship on the social organization of care work to highlight some of the implications of home care policies. I will now attempt to tie together some of the threads cutting across these micro-level examples in order to consider their macro-level implications for theory and practice.

As Mrs. Durham's case reveals, home care policies disrupt divisions of caring expertise and bring into sharp relief the problems for nursing of a professionalizing strategy that places subjective knowledge of the patient at the center of claims to jurisdiction. With the entry of family carers into health care work, subjectivities may be contested and questions asked about who really knows the patient and whose version is to prevail. I have argued that resolving these issues is not simply about melding local and global knowledge, as some writers have presumed. Family carers and health professionals come to know the cared-for person through competing interpretative frames. Despite nurses' public jurisdictional claims about a holistic approach to care, we have seen that those involved in the case of Mrs. Durham were strongly influenced by a biomedical frame. This contrasted with the perspective of Mrs. Durham, whose sense-making was undertaken within a social frame rooted in her relationship with her husband, their shared experience of illness and their life together.

Evidently any theory of home care must be able to accommodate the multiple discourses that bisect this field and develop an understanding of the processes through which they may be brought together or kept apart. There are several existing conceptual frameworks offering such a point of departure.

Strauss' (1978) social world perspective immediately springs to mind. This involves recognizing that processes of interaction involve the intersection of individuals from different social worlds or arenas. Members of a social world share commitments, resources and discourses for understanding, and when members from different social worlds come together these alignments are consequential for action. In a previously published paper from Study 1 (Allen, Griffiths, and Lyne 2004b), we drew on Elias' (1978) game theory framework to understand the interactions of the different actors involved. Because participants inhabit different social worlds, they can disagree about goals, have different priorities, perspectives and differential access to resources with which to pursue these. These differences may be overt or covert, and while negotiations between health and social care providers and families are formally constituted as cooperative occasions, interactions can be transformed into a competition or at least include competitive elements, increasing the complexity of the interaction and producing an outcome which nobody planned or could have predicted. We saw some good examples of these processes in the cases of Mrs. Durham, Edward and Rosa.

Frame analysis is another potentially useful conceptual tool. Frame analysis was introduced into the literature by Goffman (1974), and has been applied to medical practice by Dodier (1998). Dodier examines the practice of occupational medicine to reveal how doctors manage the relationship between an *administrative frame,* in which people are all the same category and treated in the same way, and a *clinical frame,* in which the doctor follows a course that leaves room for an individual's unpredictable particularities. In the case of Mrs. Durham, I have identified the operation of a 'biomedical frame' and a 'social frame' in the constitution of John's 'needs' and how framing need in different ways leads to different conclusions about action. It is likely that closer empirical inspection will reveal other available frames through which home care decisions are shaped, such as an administrative frame. Of critical importance, for current purposes, is the articulation between frames according to the dynamics of concrete activity. Dodier distinguishes between three modalities of articulation between frames: temporal succession in which the two types of framing follow each other; controversies in which debate develops between different types of framing; and a combination of forms of action in which frames coexist. In the context of home care policy, we need to focus attention on the framing of issues and the consequences this has for action.

Another cross-cutting theme in the cases considered in this chapter is the need to include in any conceptualization of the caring division of labor both its affective and its work components. In the past, social scientific analyses have intentionally downplayed the emotional components of care-giving in order to highlight the exploitative capacity of welfare policy. But this overlooks a key element vital to understanding this field. As the cases discussed in the chapter reveal, affective relationships shape caregivers' understanding of need and their willingness and ability to undertake care-giving work. Home care privileges caring relationships without acknowledging their interaction with the actual work of caring. Rather than social ties being a foundation for caring for someone, it is precisely *because* a relationship is emotionally close that caring work may be made deeply problematic.

This reinforces the arguments I have developed elsewhere about the need for the role of therapeutic relationships to be reconsidered in the context of professional nursing (Allen 2004, 2007; Dingwall and Allen 2001), as well as highlighting the requirement for greater attention to body work in nursing research. Nurses have always had a deeply ambivalent orientation to intimate caregiving: on the one hand, stressing its value, but on the other, ignoring the subject in nursing scholarship and delegating the work to unqualified carers in practice. As a consequence, public understanding of bodies and body work is limited and affective relations are assumed to be a sufficient prerequisite for caring work. This clearly reveals the dangers of an occupational strategy that has focused on subjective relationships as the foundation for caring whilst simultaneously ignoring the skills involved. As the implications of home care policies are fully realized, what is emerging is the outworking of gendered occupational strategies that emphasize the qualities and skills associated with the presumed natural talents of women. Seen through a management lens, the foregrounding of emotionally intimate relationships as the perquisite for caring provides a warrant for rationalizing services and redrawing the caring division of labor to produce marked inequalities in provision.

So where does this leave the role of nursing in the home care context? In previously published reviews of ethnographic studies of nursing work, I identified the core nursing role to be that of the healthcare intermediary (Allen 2004, 2007). The reviews were primarily based on studies of nursing in institutional settings and how far the findings might be extended to the other contexts in which nurses work is uncertain. Theoretically, home care nurses are well placed to assume the role of intermediary and play a crucial role in negotiating a space in which the frames constituting a home care situation can coexist. However, in real-life practice other pressures can lead to a privileging of one perspective over another. This brings to mind Lipsky's (1980) observations on front line worker's role in interpreting and implementing social policies in a process he describes as "street level bureaucracy." Lipsky points to the constraints within which street-level policy-making takes place and the danger that individual prejudices shape actions. His is a pessimistic portrayal of policy implementers and their effects, and our cases have shown that there is certainly empirical support for such an interpretation. Equally, however, the dilemmas and contradictions of home care policies seem to demand the exercise of discretion. As

Lipsky observes, the value of discretion is the ability to have diverse interpretations of a situation and to interpret policy as appropriate according to the circumstances at hand. We have seen how this can happen to positive effect in the case of Brian. This is why there is a need for the tensions and dilemmas shaping experiences of home care to be made explicit in order to move us towards a reconceptualization of the issues involved and to build this into policy and practice. The associated challenge is making the work involved in mediating caring work visible.

As we have seen, home care is a delicate balancing act between managing the needs of the cared-for with those of the carer and in reaching innovative solutions in order to accommodate need within the restrictions of home care policies. Here the nursing function becomes that of mediator in the management of ecologies of care-giving and the ethical challenge that of keeping in the foreground families' needs in the face of external pressures and policy constraints.

In this chapter I have drawn on selected empirical evidence to scrutinize home care policies and practice and find a way of making connections between them. These fragments have revealed the tensions and contradictions of home care for families and the challenges they present to the health professions both in policy and in practice. It seems to me that there is a role for professional caregivers in this field, but this may have a rather different shape and function to that which currently dominates public jurisdictional claims and the first task is to deepen and refine our understanding of the issues involved. I make no claims to have offered an exhaustive account here and many loose ends remain. I hope however to have provided some suggestions about how we might progress thinking in the field with the aim of stimulating debate.

REFERENCES

Allen, Davina. 2000a. "I'll tell you what suits me best if you don't mind me saying": a sociological analysis of lay participation in health care. *Nursing Inquiry* 7: 182–190.
——— 2000b. Negotiating the role of expert carers on an adult hospital ward. *Sociology of Health and Illness* 22(2): 149–171.
——— 2001. *The changing shape of nursing practice.* London: Routledge.
——— 2002a. Time and space on the hospital ward: Shaping the scope of nursing practice. In *Nursing and the division of labour in health care*, edited by Davina Allen and David Hughes, 23–52. Basingstoke: Palgrave Macmillan.
——— 2002b. Creating a participatory caring context on hospital wards. In *Nursing and the division of labour in health care*, edited by Davina Allen and David Hughes, 151–182. Basingstoke: Palgrave Macmillan.
——— 2004. Re-reading nursing and re-writing practice: towards an empirically-based reformulation of the nursing mandate. *Nursing Inquiry* 11(4): 271–283.
——— 2007. What did you do at work today? Profession-building and doing nursing. *International Nursing Review* 54(1): 41–48.
Allen, Davina, Lesley Griffiths, Patricia Lyne, Lee Monaghan and D. Murphy. 2000. *Delivering health and social care: Changing roles, responsibilities and*

relationships. Final report submitted to the Welsh Office of Research and Development for Health and Social Care.

Allen, Davina, Lesley Griffiths and Patricia Lyne. 2004a. Understanding complex trajectories in health and social care provision. *Sociology of Health and Illness* 26(7): 1008–1030.

——— 2004b. Accommodating health and social care need: routine resource allocation processes in stroke rehabilitation. *Sociology of Health and Illness* 26(4): 411–432.

Armstrong, David. 1983. The fabrication of nurse-patient relationships. *Social Science and Medicine* 17(8): 457–460.

Dingwall, Robert and Davina Allen. 2001. The implications of healthcare reforms for the profession of nursing. *Nursing Inquiry* 8(2): 64–74.

Dodier, Nicolas. 1998. Clinical practice and procedures in occupational medicine: A study of the framing of individuals. In *Differences in medicine: Unravelling practices, techniques, and bodies*, edited by Marc Berg and Annemarie Mol, 53–85. Durham and London: Duke University Press.

Elias, Norbert. 1978. *What is sociology?* London: Hutchinson.

——— 1983. *The court society*. Oxford: Basil Blackwell.

Exley, Catherine. 1999. Testaments and memories: negotiating after death-identities. *Mortality* 4(3): 226–249.

Exley, Catherine and Davina Allen. 2007. A critical examination of home care: end of life care as an illustrative case. *Social Science and Medicine* 65: 2317–2327.

Exley, Catherine and Freya Tyrer. 2005. Bereaved carers' views of a hospice at home service. *International Journal of Palliative Nursing* 11(5): 242–247.

Exley, Catherine and Gayle Letherby. 2001. Managing a disrupted life-course: issues of identity and emotional work. *Health* 5(1): 112–132.

Exley, Catherine, David Field, Linda Jones and Tim Stokes. 2005. Palliative care in the community for cancer and end-stage cardio-respiratory disease: the views of patients, lay-carers and health care professionals. *Palliative Medicine* 19: 76–83.

Finch, Janet. 1990. The politics of community care. In *Gender and caring: Work and welfare in Britain and Scandinavia*, edited by Clare Ungerson, 34–58.New York: Harvester Wheatsheaf.

Goffman, Erving. 1974. *Frame analysis: An essay on the organization of experience*. New York: Harper and Row.

Harvath, T. A., P. G. Archibold, B. J. Stewart, S. Godow, J. M. Kirshling, L. L. Miller, J. Hogan, K. Brody and J. Schook. 1994. Establishing partnerships with family caregivers: local and cosmopolitan knowledge. *Journal of Gerontological Nursing* 20: 29–35.

Henwood, Melanie. 1990. *Community care and elderly people*. London: Family Policy Studies Centre.

Lawler, Jocelyn. 1991. *Behind the screens: Nursing, somology and the problem of the body*. London: Churchill Livingstone.

Lipsky, Michael. 1980. *Street-level bureaucracy: Dilemmas of the individual in public services*. New York: Russell Sage Publications.

May, Carl. 1992. Nursing work, nurses' knowledge, and the subjectification of the patient. *Sociology of Health and Illness* 14(4): 472–487.

McKinley, Robert K., Tim Stokes, Catherine Exley and David Field. 2004. Care of people dying with malignant and cardiorespiratory disease in general practice. *British Journal of General Practice* 54: 909–913.

Nolan, Mike, Gordon Grant and John Keady. 1996. *Understanding family care*. Buckingham: Open University Press.

Parker, Gillian. 1993. *With this body: Caring and disability in marriage*. Buckingham: Open University Press.

Strauss, Anslem. 1978. A social world perspective. *Studies in Symbolic Interaction* 1(1): 119–128.

Taraborrelli, Patricia. 1994. Innocents, converts and old hands: the experiences of Alzheimer's disease caregivers. In *Qualitative studies in health and medicine*, edited by Michael Bloor and Patricia Taraborrelli, 22–42. Aldershot: Avebury.

Twigg, Julia and Karl Atkin. 1994. *Carers perceived: Policy and practice in informal care*. Buckingham: Open University Press.

6 Assisting the Frail Elderly to Live a Good Life Through Home Care Practice

Kristín Björnsdóttir

Governments in many countries have developed policies aimed at encouraging and helping the elderly and those who suffer from long-term illness to continue to live in their own homes for as long as possible. As a result of this, home care has become of key importance in welfare services of the 21st century. At the same time, home care has often been described as a contested area of practice, particularly during periods of economic retrenchment. In financially constrained environments, home care clients' needs for assistance tend to be defined as low priority and not eligible for public support. This is of particular concern to the frail elderly, who often have complex but diffuse health and social needs that call for services that must be tailored to individual circumstances. Studies from different countries have demonstrated how home care services have been restructured in such a way that opportunities to provide flexible and patient-centered care are seriously limited (Aronson 2001, 2002; Aronson and Sinding 2000; Ceci 2006a, 2006b; Ceci and Purkis 2009; Dahl and Eriksen 2005; Purkis 2001). This trend is commonly attributed to the infiltration of ideas around market-driven operations, such as managed care, in public welfare services (Aronson 2001; Björnsdóttir 2009; Dahl and Eriksen 2005). In policy documents, services are characterized by demands for standardization and a demonstration of measurable outcomes, while questions of what might constitute good and ethically valid care are often left unattended.

A number of authors draw attention to these developments and call for a radical re-thinking in relation to the way in which home care is conceptualized and provided (Aronson and Neysmith 1997; Aronson and Sinding 2000; Buhler-Wilkerson 2007; Ceci 2006a; Levine 1999). Their suggestions call for a critical analysis of home care practice. In this paper, I hope to contribute to such an analysis of what good home care for the frail elderly may look like. My analysis is based on findings from an ethnographic study conducted at a number of locations that offer public home care in a metropolitan area in Iceland. As I observed the home care nurses doing their work, I became fascinated by their ability to work with the different patients they were assigned to in a relaxed and knowledgeable manner. Later, I found much resonance between their approach and the way in which good care was theorized by a group of social scientists and philosophers (Mol 2008; Moser 2008; Pols 2004; Thygesen 2009). I will begin with a brief overview of their work, and then I will describe my study.

HOME CARE AS PRACTICE

Within the current ethos, discourses where citizens are assured entitlements to social security have been displaced with a new discourse of service users who are active, individualistic and self-interested consumers, concerned with accessing services in the market, exercising choice and seeking equality. Addressing home care practice in Canada, Ceci and Purkis (2009) pointed out how the discourses available to draw on in practice seem only to allow for a narrow understanding of what this practice is about. In theoretical articulation of practice and policy documents, both practitioners and clients tend to be described as rational, autonomous decision makers. This view of practice discounts the complex contextual issues that shape daily life and the relationship between practitioners and patients and does not acknowledge the political nature of the situation (Purkis 2001).

On a similar note, Mol (2008, 2009) pointed out how the care of people with long-term illnesses has increasingly been framed based on what she identified as the logic of choice. In this logic, patients are portrayed as rational decision makers, weighing the costs and benefits of the different ways to respond to a given illness. Within this logic, the role of professionals is to present alternatives for consideration, while it is up to the patients to decide what alternative they choose. Mol suggests that it might be helpful to shift attention from the cognitive processes involved in decision making to the everyday practice of living with a particular condition. Then rather than studying the patient's decisions or choices, we might explore the extent to which they are able to adapt suggested treatments to their situation and organize their daily life, taking their ability and condition into consideration. Such an understanding of practice demands knowledge of context and the constellations of humans and technologies that may aid in sustaining the person being cared for (Thygesen 2009), and an exploration of ideals and values that the workers espouse (Pols 2004).

If practice is understood this way, then it could be said that professionals work with patients in formulating possible solutions and trying them out. By attending to how the context of everyday life may facilitate or prevent certain activities, we can better understand what is helpful to patients. Mol refers to this approach to practice as the logic of care. Clinical work, in this logic, focuses on the nature of care that each person needs and wishes for, rather than aiming at particular pre-determined standards. What is needed is often far from clear at the beginning, but emerges as treatments are tried out and realized in practice.

When practice is based on the logic of care, the help provided is thought through and organized with the patient and in collaboration between care workers and relatives. New ways are tried out and re-evaluated until a suitable approach has been found; this, Mol refers to as doctoring. What may suit one person may not be helpful for another and what may work at one time but may not work next time. Good clinical work is experimental and inventive. It "attunes to the complex particularities of a specific patient in his or her specific circumstances" (Struhkamp, Mol and Swierstra 2009, 71–72). The logic of care does not impose guilt, but calls for tenacity, for a sticky combination of adaptability and perseverance (Mol 2008).

The logic of care focuses on the practicalities of everyday life rather than rational decision making or people's account of living with a particular disease. Therefore, studying practice from this perspective calls for an ethnographic approach, which provides an opportunity to observe caring as it is enacted in real-life situations. A number of authors have recently conducted such studies in different care settings, attempting to describe what constitutes good care. For example, Moser (2008) described how the nursing staff on a unit for Alzheimer patients tried to understand the patients' ways of expressing themselves despite the patients' inability to articulate their needs and wishes clearly. This often demanded reading non-verbal cues, facial expressions and body language. The nurses related to the patients and the situation 'here and now', trying to keep the communication clear and simple. In another study on a unit for individuals with dementia, the focus was practices involved in the intake of food and drink. The authors pointed out the complex ways in which the staff tried to adapt what was being offered in response to the various needs and wishes among the patients (Harbers, Mol and Stollmeyer 2002). Food and drink are media for care and satisfy longings and customs. By studying the practicalities and materialities of daily care, the modes of giving food and drink in this case, the authors tried to understand what might constitute good care on a unit and what was being striven for and what was avoided.

The study of home care presented here is similar to the above studies in that it was an ethnographic study of home care practice. At the time the data collection took place, home care in Iceland had not been influenced by the economic discourse and the resultant rationalization and standardization of services described in many other countries. Therefore, Iceland may have been said to provide "conditions of possibility" in fostering good practices in home care (May and Purkis 1995), which I will try to tease out in this paper.

LONG-TERM CARE AT HOME IN ICELAND

Home care has traditionally been part of health care services in Iceland. When the *Act on Services for the Elderly* was initially passed in 1983, it stated that the elderly are entitled to comprehensive home care services around the clock (Act on the Elderly 1983). Home health care is part of the state-run health care services and is provided free of charge, while social services are organized by the municipalities at some cost to the users. Anyone can apply for services. However the use of home care was not widespread until the first decade of the 21st century. The tradition in Iceland has been that when need for assistance with daily life increased, the elderly person applied for placement in a nursing home. The media has primarily discussed difficulties and insecurity faced by the elderly and people with long-term conditions in relation to lack of available placements in nursing homes. It was only very recently that interest in home care services became noticeable among policy makers and spokespersons for the elderly. In policy documents (Ministry of Health and Social Services 2003, 2006), in the media and in statements issued by lobby groups representing the elderly, the disabled and the chronically ill, the home is now identified as the optimal place of living for citizens as they age.

Little attention has been paid to home care services in research, but in recent policy documents home care was described as underdeveloped. For example, a study by the Icelandic National Audit Office (2005) concluded that home care was haphazardly organized in different parts of the country. The level and comprehensiveness of home care services varied on a large scale between municipalities, and the integration between health and social services was often found lacking. These findings raised concerns since, by national law, all citizens are entitled to comparable services. One of the main obstacles to the development of comprehensive home care services has been an undeveloped organizational structure and unclear responsibility for service provision. Another major complaint has been the poor coordination between health care and social services (Magnúsdóttir 2006).

Method

Using an ethnographic approach (Hammersley and Atkinson 1995), the focus of this study was the everyday life of the frail elderly receiving home care and the enactment of practices by official service workers, nurses in this case, aimed at providing assistance. Practice was understood pragmatically and seen as "an intensely grounded activity that takes place between bodies" (May and Purkis 1995, 289), as the coming together of the practitioner and the person being cared for in a mutual exchange, where both parties bring their knowledge and understanding (Purkis 2003). Through such an exchange, the identity of participants is constantly being accomplished. Understood this way, practice is neither set nor predictable, rational or linear, but rather dynamic and invested with power.

The ethnographic approach calls for an understanding of practice as social rather than bio-medical and demands attention to the impact of context. Latimer's (1997, 2000, 2003) study is an interesting example of how 'the social' influences the care of the frail elderly in the emergency room at a university hospital in the UK. By observing how nurses cared for elderly patients in an acute care hospital, she was able to identify contradictory agendas, as she describes:

> Critically, I trace what and who authorises the flow of materials to and from the bedside. It is in these accounts that one can find what has authority, what gives permission to privilege one kind of work or one kind of patient over another. (2003, 238)

In the study presented here, home care was explored through fieldwork and formal interviews with elderly individuals who needed considerable assistance with daily activities and who lived in their own homes. Relatives or friends who provided help and the nurses who organized the public services were also interviewed.

Settings and Data Collection

At the time of the data collection for this study, health care services were organized and administered by the state, while social services were the responsibility of the municipalities. Therefore, home nursing care was organized by state-run community health centers. The catchment area of each center varied, but in most of them, the group of patients receiving home care was small. This led to difficulties in providing services around the clock and on weekends. A few months after the data collection started, the decision was made to unite the home care nursing services in Reykjavik in one center. In the neighboring municipalities, home care nursing continued to be organized by the local community centers.

Permission to conduct the study was given by the Icelandic Ethical Review Board, and collaboration was established with a number of health care centers in Reykjavik and vicinity. The directors of the community health centers were contacted, and where collaboration was agreed upon, the director was asked to suggest households that fit the research criteria. When a decision had been made to include the household in the data collection, the nurses at the center contacted the client and/or family to ask them to participate in the study.

The first part of the data collection took place at different community centers in Reykjavik and neighboring municipalities, but the latter part was located at the larger, amalgamated home nursing center. The data collection was designed around cases which were defined as individual households in which one member needed assistance with performing activities of daily life due to age, illness or disability. Before contacting individuals in a household being considered for participation, a nurse brought a letter of introduction and inquired about willingness to participate. Some families were not ready to participate, explaining that they were tired of intrusion into their private life, but overall, people were interested in joining the study. The data collection usually started with an interview with the client receiving home care services. In some of the households chosen, the client could not participate in an interview (due to cognitive impairment), which meant that the data comprised field notes and interviews with a relative and a nurse. At this point, the home care nurses were contacted and asked for permission to have the researcher shadow them during a home care visit. In most cases, I joined the nurse on morning rounds that lasted from 8:00 until 12:00. A relative was also contacted and asked to participate in an interview. Some of the patients did not identify a relative, which meant that in their experience, all the assistance that they needed was provided by the official sector. Finally, the nurse was interviewed. Some of the participants were interviewed a second time. All the interviews were transcribed, and fieldnotes were written after each visit.

The data were analyzed and interpreted in light of the overall study goals, focusing on the needs of the patients and the practices that had developed around their care. Particular attention was paid to the way in which the work was shared by the nurses, the relatives and the patients. Initially, each case was read and re-read to identify the work that was organized to help the person to live as good a life as was possible at home. The views and understandings of the different actors in the situation were analyzed. When the interviews and the field notes had been studied, issues started to emerge.

GOING FROM HOUSE TO HOUSE

In the first phase of my field study, I spent time with the RNs and auxiliary nurses and went with them on their rounds. I usually met with them at their workplace, where they started the shift by going over their cards and trying to figure out what might be the best way to organize the work. When describing the shift, they usually talked about tasks that needed to be done during each visit, but sometimes they referred to patients who needed visits for encouragement and general support. They described how things tended to change fast and that they never knew what to expect. Often they were asked to do an extra visit to a new patient who had just been added or to respond to an emergency situation. All the RNs and auxiliary nurses had mobile phones which they used for contact, co-ordination and to make arrangements with the patients, but the phones were also used to re-direct their work when something came up. They usually had to work fast to be able to visit all the patients that they were responsible for.

On one of my morning rounds, I followed Lilja, an RN working in a community center close to Reykjavik. Our visits took us to different homes in the neighborhood, small apartments and single houses. Most of the homes were well kept, but some were run down and had not been cleaned recently. We came into different homes that reflected the background, personal style and abilities of the patients. Many of them had a picture of the place where they were born and had grown up hanging prominently over the sofa or in the entrance of their home. Most homes also had family pictures on display, which provided an obvious opportunity for the nurses to become familiar with the support network and social relationships. Some of the patients lived alone, but others lived with a relative, usually a spouse. This is a quote[1] from the field notes:

> We started by seeing Gudrun, an elderly woman who lives in a sheltered housing apartment in a new building complex. Lilja rang the doorbell, but then she took out a key and let us in. She called out, "It is only the home care nurse," and someone responded, "Is it you, my dear Lilja?" The apartment was small, and everything was conveniently arranged. There were many family pictures on the walls and hand-embroidered pillows on the sofa. Lilja introduced me, and we both took off our coats and shoes, but then she and Gudrun went into the bathroom, where Lilja helped her with some medication and to wash and get dressed. When they came out of the bathroom, Lilja helped Gudrun to put on a blouse. Gudrun asked me to help with the buttons. While doing so, I commented on the family pictures, and Gudrun told me about her children and grandchildren. (Kristin Björnsdóttir, fieldnotes from community center 3)

In many ways, this was a typical visit I observed when following the nurses who were working at the community centers. The atmosphere was relaxed and casual, and the discussions shifted back and forth between a social and bio-medical level. The nurses seemed to know their patients' situations quite well. In conversations that we had between visits, they often told me about difficulties that patients were facing and how they tried to help.

After Gudrun, we went to see a number of elderly people in the same building, one man who had chronic foot wounds related to diabetes, another with complications from heart failure and one woman with beginning dementia. Then we drove to a number of different locations in the neighborhood. Lilja dressed wounds, gave shots, performed physical assessments such as blood pressure measurements and brought pre-packed medications to the patients. On a few visits, there were complicated emotional issues to attend to. As she went about doing whatever she came to do, Lilja often brought up discussions around some worries that the patient had had in previous visits. She asked the people how they were doing, and then she turned to whatever task had brought her. In most cases, the visit was uncomplicated in that nothing unexpected turned up.

In their work, the nurses I observed tried to attend to the preferences that were articulated by the patients or their relatives. Their focus was on the needs and wishes of the patients. Their practice seemed to be in line with what Mol articulated in her idea around the logic of care: attentive, flexible and imaginative.

It is Their Territory: Doing Home Care

All the nurses that I shadowed and who participated in the interviews mentioned that going into people's homes made home care nursing very different from nursing in health care institutions. "You are there on their territory," they would say. That meant that you respected their ways of living, such as their preferences for bedtime, personal cleanliness and tidiness. One nurse described the situation in this way:

> When I work as a home care nurse, I am working in the patient's territory. It is their space where they feel safe. This is different from the hospital environment where patients seem to hand themselves over to the staff. At home, they have much more to say. (Björnsdóttir, interview with nurse)

It was both challenging and rewarding for the nurses to understand the lived reality of the patients. They explained how they tried to provide care that helped patients address the difficulties that they were enduring. Part of this respect for patients' preferences was the different ways in which the nurses related to the patients. Some patients greeted the nurses as friends and offered them coffee. They also told the nurses about what had happened since they last visited and asked them about their situation. The nurses participated in these conversations while they went about doing whatever it was the patient needed, and if time allowed, they might have a cup of coffee. Other patients said little, indicating that they were not interested in conversation and would appreciate a quick stop. As one night nurse explained to me, "I have helped Pall going to bed in the evening for many years, and I am not sure that he even knows my name."

This variation in the way in which the nurses practiced was often not based on discussions with the patients, but resulted from their reading of the situation. This was similar to the description by Pols (2005), one of Mol's associates, based on her observations of practical situations where care was provided to patients on long-term psychiatric wards. Many of them did not express their views or preferences directly but used non-verbal ways of indicating their wishes. Pols referred to this as enacting appreciation, which means "making known what they like or dislike by verbal or non-verbal means in a given material environment, in situations that are co-produced by others" (203). This situation is co-produced in that it is dependent on interaction with others—nurses in this case—and the material world. As Pols explained, "being aware of the ways in which patients enact their appreciation can show how they live specific and diverse daily lives with the people and objects around them" (215).

Flexible Organizational Structures

The approach used by the nurses described above was supported by the organizational structure at the community health centers. The work group was small and collaboration among the workers seemed to be good, although there were exceptions. What was striking was the freedom that the RNs and LPNs had to organize the work as they thought best. There were no re-imbursement schemes for the services, and in the initial phase of the fieldwork, there were no guidelines regarding the work that was expected of each worker. This changed, but the nurses continued to do errands that might not be on the list, such as taking the trash out on their way. In some instances, they even went to the store for groceries. During the interviews, I asked the RNs to describe their work. This is how Dora responded:

> Well, we are constantly re-evaluating how we work, making new plans. You wonder if you can make fewer visits, or if you need to have them more frequently. Usually, we start by going rather often, particularly if we detect some difficulties such as depression or strained relationships in the home. When we feel that a rapport has been made and that trust has developed, we can decrease the number of visits. (Björnsdóttir, interview with nurse)

It was striking to observe how the nurses seemed to understand their work differently from home care nurses in many other countries where complex rules have been developed around service eligibility and advanced administrative structures for accounting for the work. The nurses observed here based the organization of the care primarily on their own discretion of what might be the most helpful and beneficial way of providing care. In informal interviews during the fieldwork and in formal interviews, both the RNs and the LPNs described how they discussed the best way to provide assistance with the resources available. As an example, they took turns at going to the patients who needed frequent visits. Each had their day, which meant that rather than going daily, they would make a visit once a week or every third or fourth day. This was done in situations where the care was physically and emotionally demanding, and the intent was to prevent emotional exhaustion. By sharing the burden of difficult care situations, they felt better equipped to help.

Admittedly, the nurses who participated in the interviews varied in their enthusiasm and motivation in relation to their job. Some said that they had initially started to work in home care because of their personal situation, but not because of direct interest in this area of practice. For a single mother with young children, the work allowed for some flexibility in attending to the children, popping home to see that everything was going fine between visits, and so on. As they learned about the work more, they had started to enjoy it. Most of them said that they liked home care, that they enjoyed meeting different people and felt that they were able to provide assistance. This was what many of them saw as the most important facet of their job. As one said, "I get my kick out of knowing how to navigate the system and being able to find solutions."

Difficulties in Accomplishing What Needs to be Done

What discouraged and frustrated the nurses was having no solutions or being unable to obtain the help that people needed. In some situations no-one was willing to take responsibility for a particular patient group, which meant that they were between systems. Both the nurses and the relatives described how they spent a lot of time on the phone, trying to get an answer regarding a request for services such as day care or respite care. This was experienced very negatively by the nurses.

Although many of the GPs made an effort to keep the co-operation between themselves and the home care nurses strong by trying to respond quickly when home care nurses contacted them, sometimes no response was given, which frustrated the nurses. Most GPs did not make house calls, which meant that when the patient was deemed by the nurse to require medical attention, the nurses had to call an ambulance to get the patient to the emergency room for a thorough medical examination. This was very frustrating for them, and it was also looked upon negatively by the hospital. The following quote from a field note gives an example of the difficulties encountered by a nurse.

> We went to visit Rosa, an 82-year-old woman who has been diagnosed with beginning Alzheimer. Rosa lives alone. Her apartment was beautifully arranged and impeccable, as was she herself, nicely groomed and gracious in her movements and expressions. Anna brought a new stack of pre-packed medicine and asked her how she was doing. She said that the problem with her urine was disturbing her. Anna did not respond to that initially, but Rosa was persistent. She said to Anna that this was bothersome, made her feel unclean and that she smelled. Then Anna started to ask specific questions related to incontinence, when she was not able to get to the bathroom and how often, if there was a lot of urine that she lost, etc. She said that she would look into it. On our way out to the car, Lilja told me that she would call Rosa's daughter and try to get her involved. She also told me that it was difficult to get the GPs to write a prescription for pads because they were having some sort of fight with the Ministry of Health over how that was reimbursed. (Björnsdóttir, fieldnotes)

This was only one of many examples where the nurses were not able to accomplish what they saw as being of central importance in assisting the patients and their relatives. In such situations, they described themselves as unable to impact the situation. This was something beyond them.

When Preference and Practice Do Not Match

Although the nurses said that they tried to organize their services around the needs and wishes of the patients and their caregivers, complaints related to the services were raised in a number of interviews both by patients and their relatives. Dissatisfaction related to timing of assistance such as being helped to go to bed and handing out medications. Many of the younger people made these complaints but in general, elderly patients said that they were pleased with the services they received. However, their relatives commented on the timing of the distribution of evening medications such as sleeping pills, which they thought were handed out too early. Some of the patients and their spouses mentioned that the nurses were often in a rush when they came on their rounds and did not provide enough time for discussion. As one woman said, "It is just in and out, and they are gone before you can open your mouth." One participant, an elderly man with a foot wound that needed dressing every day, said in an interview, "I need to eat and take my medication before they do the wound dressing. That takes me about half an hour, and that is why I prefer that they come around 9:30. Sometimes they will come just after eight, and that is awful." Interestingly, the nurse later commented on this in our interview, saying that she had arrived at this man's place early one morning and did not know about his need to have breakfast before the wound change. She said that she had to wait for him while he was eating breakfast, commenting that he has all kinds of ceremonies: "first a spoonful of cod liver oil and then cereal and followed by some fruit and finally the medications."

The flexibility that characterized the organizational structure raised the danger of unreliability and that the visits might be organized around the nurses' personal needs and preferences. It may be speculated that the way in which the work was organized and the lack of rules meant that each worker could influence the pace of the work, sometimes prioritizing her personal situation outside of work. By working fast, the nurses were, for example, able to get off work early and attend to whatever things they might need to do personally. This meant that sometimes they were more hurried and brisk than the time allowed for visits demanded.

In some respects, the nurses were also uncritical about traditions that had been established and that they followed. As an example, although they themselves took a bath every morning, assistance with bathing was only provided once a week. This was not discussed among the nurses but patients and particularly relatives mentioned this rule as insufficient. A daughter said: "My mother is diabetic and she sweats a lot and should have a bath more often than once a week." It was also noticeable that when co-operation with relatives was needed the nurses tended to call the women among them.

DISCUSSION

In her book on the logic of care, Mol (2008) challenges health care professionals to think about ways in which they can help their patients to a more livable existence. This means being thoughtful about each situation and trying to understand the impact of the context, understanding the help provided by relatives, being aware of how different biographies impact the people involved and how their financial situation and the resources available in the community support living. By listening to what the patient and his or her relatives have to say about life, the care worker can design services that support and facilitate the life wished for.

In many ways, the nurses observed and interviewed in this study shared this understanding of practice. Being able to help and find solutions to the problems that had a negative impact on the wellbeing of the elderly patients was their main goal. At some of the community health centers, the nurses had developed a collective understanding of their practice and organized the care in an innovative and flexible way. This approach was facilitated by the limited structure and regulations imposed. In their understanding, decisions around the provision of care were in their hands.

There is usually a downside to everything. In this case, the organizational flexibility allowed the nurses to move their work around to better suit their personal schedule, sometimes at the expense of the comfort and preferences of the patients. Although the younger patients did raise objections, the elderly did not do so. It was their relatives who pointed out that it would be more convenient to, say, help their parents to bed later in the evening. This situation needs further exploration, but this seemed to happen in work settings where the cohesiveness of the work group was weak and where the work ideals had not been discussed to any great extent. In her study of good care on long-term psychiatric units, Pols (2004, 2008) explored the ideals that the workers espoused. She refers to her analysis as empirical ethics, which was reflected in the way in which good care was shaped in daily activities, events and routines on wards for patients with long-term psychiatric illnesses. As Pols points out, ideals of good care develop in time and new ideals replace old. New ideals such as 'person-centered care' or 'patient autonomy' are often imported from theoretical literature, but then they develop further and are adapted to practice. By exploring what patients see as bothersome and what might be helpful, ideals around care take shape. Such an exploration demands a critical reflection among the staff. In the community centers where the staff had well-developed ideals that were enacted in practice, as was described above, such reflection took place at staff meetings and in informal conversations in the field. The flexibility in the way in which the services were organized, the limited use of standardized work methods and the general tendency to be active all seemed to enhance such an approach.

The logic of care as theorized by Mol (2008) is characterized by striving for improvements in the patient's life. She points out that rather than attempting to prove which interventions are most effective, we might want to develop studies to explore how they work and how they can be improved (Mol 2006). As she points out, treatments fit people in different ways and what may be helpful and important for one patient may be of little comfort to another. Therefore, there may not be a best or most effective way to treat a particular condition, but a number of ways. Moser's (2010) study of advanced dementia care is one such example. By studying and articulating the practices used by the staff, she was able to draw out the aspects of care that are of particular importance. As she points out, a head nurse on one of the wards used a video camera to document the ways in which the staff approached the patients. She organized sessions with the staff where they looked at and discussed excerpts from the recording, which highlighted particular practices. These typically highlighted the capacities for caring that reflected its embodied and choreographed nature.

In this paper, I highlighted some aspects of home care practice that I identified as important to good care. Of particular importance was the way in which the flexible organizational structure allowed the staff to explore and respond to each patient's needs and wishes. At the same time, the flexibility became a threat to quality care if the workers had not developed clear ideals. I hope that these findings can be useful in supporting important practices in home care. I also think that the ideas brought up by the authors cited here, such as the importance of creating opportunities to spend time together to discuss the care of the patients, are of great importance.

NOTES

1. Interviews translated from Icelandic by the author.

REFERENCES

Act on the Elderly. 1983. Reykjavik: The Icelandic parliament.

Anderson, Magdalena, Ingalill Rahm Hallberg and Anna Karin Edberg. 2008. Old people receiving municipal care, their experiences of what constitutes a good life in the last phase of life: a qualitative study. *International Journal of Nursing Studies* 45(6): 818–828.

Aronson, Jane. 2001. Frail and disabled users of home care: confident consumers or disentitled citizens? *Canadian Journal of Aging* 21(1): 11–25.

——— 2002. Elderly people's account of home care rationing: missing voices in long-term care policy debates. *Ageing and Society* 22: 399–418.

Aronson, Jane and Sheila M. Neysmith. 1997. The retreat of the state and long-term care provision: implication for frail elderly people, unpaid family careers and paid home care workers. *Studies in Political Economy* 53: 37–66.

Aronson, Jane and Chris Sinding. 2000. Home care users' experiences of fiscal constraint: challenges and opportunities for case management. *Care Management Journals* 2(4): 220–225.

Björnsdóttir, Kristín. 2009. The ethics and politics of home care. *International Journal of Nursing Studies* 46: 732–739.

Buhler-Wilkerson, Karen. 2007. Care of the chronically ill at home: an unresolved dilemma in health policy for the United States. *The Milbank Quarterly* 85(4): 611–639.

Ceci, Christine. 2006a. "What she says she needs doesn't make a lot of sense": seeing and knowing in a field study of home-care case management. *Nursing Philosophy* 7: 90–99.

——— 2006b. Impoverishment of practice: analysis of effects of economic discourses in home care case management practice. *Canadian Journal of Nursing Leadership* 19 (1): 56–68.

Ceci, Christine and Mary Ellen Purkis. 2009. Bridging gaps in risk discourse: home care case management and clinical choices. *Sociology of Health and Illness* 31(2): 201–214.

Dahl, Hanne Marline and Tine Rask Eriksen. 2005. *Dilemmas of care in the Nordic welfare state*. Hants: Ashgate.

Hammersley, Martyn and Paul Atkinson. 1995. *Ethnography: Principles in practice*. 2nd ed. London: Routledge.

Harbers, Hans, Annemarie Mol and Alice Stollmeyer. (2002). Food matters: arguments for an ethnography of daily care. *Theory, Culture and Society* 19(5/6): 207–226.

Icelandic National Audit Office. 2005. *Þjónusta við aldraða: Stjórnsýsluúttekt* (Services for the elderly). Reykjavik: Icelandic National Audit Office.

Latimer, Joanna. 1997. Giving patients a future: the constituting of classes in an acute medical unit. *Sociology of Health & Illness* 19(2): 160–185.

———. 2000. *The conduct of care: understanding nursing practice*. Oxford: Blackwell Science.

——— 2003. Studying the women in white. In *Advanced qualitative research for nursing,* edited by Joanna Latimer, 231–246. Oxford: Blackwell.

Levine, Carol. 1999. Home sweet hospital: the nature and limits of private responsibilities for home health care. *Journal of Aging and Health* 11(3): 341–359.

May, Carl and Mary Ellen Purkis. 1995. The configuration of nurse-patient relationships: a critical view. *Scholarly Inquiry for Nursing Practice,* 9(4): 283–295.

Magnúsdóttir, Berglind. 2006. *Samþætting heimaþjónusta í Reykjavík—febrúar 2004 til febrúar 2006* (Integration of home care in Reykjavik—February 2004 to February 2006). Reykjavik: The City of Reykjavik and Primary Health Care of the Capital Area—Home Nursing Centre.

Ministry of Health and Social Services. 2003. *Skýrsla stýrihóps um stefnumótun í málefnum aldraðra til ársins 2015* (Report of steering group on policies in geriatric care until 2015). Reykjavik: Ministry of Health and Social Services.

——— 2006. Ný sýn—nýjar leiðir: Áherslur heilbrigðis- og tryggingamálaráðherra í öldrunarmálum (New visions—new methods: Minister of Health and Social Services' emphases in elderly care). Reykjavík: Ministry of Health and Social Services.

Mol, Annemarie. 1999. *Body multiple: Ontology in medical practice*. Durham: Duke University Press.

——— 2006. Proving or improving: on health care research as a form of self-reflection. *Qualitative Health Research* 16(3): 405–414.

——— 2008. *The logic of care: Health and the problem of patient choice*. London: Routledge.

———— 2009. Living with diabetes: care beyond choice and control. *The Lancet* 373(9677): 1756–1757.

Moser, Ingunn. 2008. Making Alzheimer's disease matter. Enacting, interfering and doing politics of nature . *Geoforum* 39(1): 98–110.

———— 2010. Perhaps tears should not be counted but wiped away: On quality and improvement in dementia care. In *Care in practice: On tinkering in clinics, homes and farms*, edited by Annemarie Mol, Ingunn Moser and Jeanette Pols, 277–300. Bielefeld: transcript Verlag.

Pols, Jeanette. 2004. Good care: Enacting complex ideal in long-term psychiatry. PhD diss., Utrect: Trimbos-instituut.

———— 2005. Enacting appreciations: eeyond the patient perspective. *Health Care Analysis* 13(3): 203–221.

———— 2008. Which empirical research, whose ethics? Articulating ideals in long term mental health care. In *Empirical Ethics in Psychiatry*, edited by Guy Widdershoven, John Mcmillan, Tony Hope and Lieke van der Scheer, 51–68. Oxford: Oxford University Press.

Purkis, Mary Ellen. 2001. Managing home nursing care: visibility, accountability and exclusion. *Nursing Inquiry* 8(3): 141–150.

———— 2003. Moving nursing practice: Integrating theory and method. In *Advanced qualitative research for nursing,* edited by Joanna Latimer, 32–52. Oxford: Blackwell.

Struhkamp, Rita, Annemarie Mol and Tsjalling Swierstra. 2009. Dealing with in/ dependence: doctoring in physical rehabilitation practice. *Science, Technology and Human Values* 34(1): 55–76.

Thygesen, Hilde. 2009. *Technology and good dementia care: A study of technology and ethics in everyday care practice.* Oslo: Faculty of Social Sciences, Oslo University.

Part III

Practices

7 Who Can Be Against Quality?

A New Story About Home-Based Care: NPM and Governmentality

Hanne Marlene Dahl

SETTING THE SCENE

Within the last two decades, the field of elderly care in Denmark, as in the rest of the Nordic countries, has experienced major reorganizations inspired by the ideas of New Public Management (NPM). In NPM the political focus was upon efficiency, changing recently into a concern with the quality of care. Major reforms related to this drive for quality have been implemented, such as compulsory standards of quality for the municipalities (1999) and, for service users, the free choice of provider (2003). Quality was seen to be improved through the citizen's free choice between providers of home-based care—private and public. This in turn required the introduction of a provider-performer model where the estimation of needs was split off from the concrete production of care. This new story of the state as concerned with quality contains a new rationality with a strong seductive force. Quality signifies the laudable and lasting, and it becomes impossible to be against quality.

New Public Management is a transnational, dynamic and complex discourse stressing the need for the marketization of services and the use of management techniques by the state that stress professional leadership, self-engineering and self-motivation (Andersen 2001; Hood 1991; Marcussen 2002; Sahlin-Andersson 2002). Another, broader term often applied to some of the same phenomena is that of 'neo-liberalism' denoting a form of political-economic governance premised on the extension of market relationships, individualization and responsibility into all areas of life (Larner 2000). For reasons of simplicity, I will use the concept of NPM in this chapter. NPM is a complex discourse fusing two different streams of ideas and developing over time. The two streams are neo-liberal economics, and the other, a managerial stream having its origin in management studies (Hood 1991). Whereas the neo-liberal economic logic sees the introduction of markets and choice as a solution to the ills of the state, the managerial logic stresses a new understanding of leadership as the solution. The two streams of thought play out in varying ways and result in different translations of NPM in different, national contexts (Greve 2003; Schmidt 2002), but they also translate in different versions in different policy fields and levels of the state, as well as embody potential conflicts within NPM.

Whereas New Zealand and the UK have been described as frontrunners in the introduction of NPM, the Nordic countries have been seen as laggards (Christensen and Lægreid 2007). This is, amongst other things, due to the less favorable institutional context for NPM reforms in the Nordic countries due to equality being a key value (Christensen and Lægreid 2007). In whatever translation, NPM is bound to co-exist with already established values and thus can be seen as involved in an institutional layering of rationalities and values (Thelen 2000). In this respect NPM shapes the present and the future identities of home helpers and recipients of care in Denmark—a context that still provides generous and universal elderly care (Rausch 2008; Szebehely 2003). Home helpers in Denmark have traditionally been employed and trained by the state, and their occupation regulated by the state. The state discourse constructs the ideal home helper as a particular subject who requires formal training for one or one and a half years, which simultaneously inscribes her in a discourse of professionalism (Dahl 2000, 2005a). Comparatively, Danish home helpers have had a high degree of autonomy when assessing the needs of the recipients (Knijn and Verhagen 2003). However, autonomy has decreased with the introduction of the provider-performer model.

The dynamic, multifaceted and co-opting character of NPM has ensured its continued dominance (Christensen and Lægreid 2002; Clarke and Newman 1997). Whereas some have written an obituary of NPM (Dunleavy et al. 2005), others have argued that NPM is still alive, middle-aged and producing paradoxes (Hood and Peters 2004). There is an agreement in the literature that NPM is alive in a revised version (Christensen and Lægreid 2007), including in Denmark (Hansen 2008). Here we are currently experiencing struggles about NPM—both from below (Dahl 2009) and from above, as will be shown shortly.

In the mainstream literature, NPM is often seen from the perspective of organizational reform and considered in terms of its democratic implications (see for example Christensen and Lægreid 2007). Gender perspectives on neo-liberalism or NPM are often absent and feminist research has attempted to correct this bias in various ways (Knijn and Verhagen 2003; Outshoorn and Kantola 2007; Vabø 2006). However, feminist researchers studying paid and/or professional caregivers have too often identified NPM with standardization or marketization (Knijn and Verhagen 2003), neglecting the complexity and seductive character of NPM—not unlike most mainstream analyses of neo-liberalism and NPM that have underestimated the significance and complexity of this new way of thinking (Larner 2000). In this chapter I will therefore investigate how NPM, as a complex discourse in a socio-democratic welfare regime, produces new identities for those performing care, with a digression into how the discourse produces new identities for elderly people as well. The discursive changes in the understandings of elderly people have been the subject of another article of mine, where I identified a new concern with the self of the elderly, his or her development in an active and self-determining life (Dahl 2005b).

The production of new identities for the home helpers is investigated applying feminist discourse analysis (Bacchi 1999; Eveline and Bacchi 2005) and a feminist theory of recognition (Fraser 2003). Discourse analysis helps identify the argumentative logics that produce the seductiveness of a given discourse, but such analysis risks lapsing into relativism—this is avoided by introducing a critical anchoring point with a theory of recognition. Feminist discourse analysis and feminist theory of recognition help analyze the material from a critical gender perspective, i.e., whether the NPM discourses are enabling or constraining the recognition of care by state organized and paid home help.

New Public Management can be studied in various ways (Greve 2003; Larner 2000). In my study I see it as a new discourse about publicly provided care, e.g., a new story being told about care and the identities of those involved (Laclau and Mouffe 1985). It is also a discourse which represents a new art of governing, governmentality, that no longer exclusively relies on laws but instead rules through the professions and the strategic application of their scientific knowledge (Foucault 1991; Johnson 1995). More specifically, governmentality governs through the formation of ideals such as self-governance and self-reflexivity (Dean 1999).

I studied the development of NPM through examining the politico-administrative texts for the period 1996–2006 in the field of elderly care in Denmark, with a particular attention to three analytical focus points: the articulation of and struggle about care, governing and the identities of the home helpers, and the consequences of the recognition and misrecognition of the care-giving work of home helpers.

This chapter begins by presenting the theoretical framework of recognition. This is followed by a second section presenting the methodology of the study. The third section presents current developments in the Danish version of NPM in elderly care as a move towards quality and outlines the two forms this has taken. The fourth section identifies the changes and struggles about care, governing and identities. The fifth section identifies the implications of NPM for the recognition and misrecognition of home helpers. The final section concludes.

RECOGNITION

Status differentials are increasingly illegitimate in the postmodern world (Fraser 2003) and provide a catalyst for struggles for equality such as seen in sexual, ethnic and linguistic struggles (Taylor 1994; Young 1990), as well as in struggles about care (Dahl 2009). The American philosopher Nancy Fraser (1997, 2003) understands equality in social status in terms of recognition. Status equality is achieved when institutionalized patterns of cultural value constitute social actors as *peers*, capable of participating on a par with one another in social life (Fraser 2003, 29). In other words, recognition means being seen, heard (Thompson 2006) and taken into account in social interaction. Recognition is in Bauman's words a "claim to humanity" (Bauman 2001). Recognition is characteristic of a situation where a group and its work is visible (being spoken about), respected (of equal worth) and assigned prestige (receiving a positive, cultural valorization). In contrast to recognition, misrecognition is identified by silence, dominance and stereotypical representations, for example the degrading representations of the knowledge base required for good care. Such misrecognition is illustrated in the following, hypothetical statement: 'Anybody can perform care'. Fraser does not envision recognition as a final, authentic self to be reached, but sees recognition as contextually informed by struggles for recognition that are ongoing, mutable and multifaceted creations (Tully 2000, 479). Focusing upon recognition inevitably means neglecting the other two perspectives in Fraser's theoretical framework.[1]

Recognition can take place in different institutional spheres (Honneth 1994), such as the intimate sphere of the family/friends, the state and the social sphere. Within the Nordic welfare state regimes(s), the state plays a major role in structuring society and with its large involvement in care, it becomes pertinent to study it from a perspective of recognition. Studying state discourse from a perspective of recognition implies analyzing patterns of the cultural valorizations present or non-present in these texts. Whereas Fraser's earlier work suffered from a blind spot on the role of the state and its relationship to other institutions (Feldman 2002; Hobson 2003), she has in her recent work sought to remedy this neglect (Fraser 2003, 2008). Feminist state theorists have disagreed about the role of the state, seeing it as either potentially women friendly (Hernes 1987) or patriarchal (Hirdman 1994). It consequently becomes important to study whether NPM-inspired state discourses produce recognition (the women-friendly state) or misrecognition of home helpers (the patriarchal state).

DISCOURSE—AND FEMINIST DISCOURSE ANALYSIS

Framings matter. The ways socio-political problems are framed or discussed have an impact upon potential lines of argument, legitimate positions and solutions (Verloo and Lombardo 2007). Here I apply a discourse analysis inspired by Laclau and Mouffe (1985) and Bacchi (1999), where I broadly focus upon the creation of meaning, ambiguity and silence (Dahl 2000). Meaning refers to the identification of discursive horizons (relations of meaning), silence (absence of speech) and ambiguity (identification of eventual competing logics). Silence is that which is left un- problematized or disappears out of the texts as something that cannot be spoken about

(Bacchi 1999; Whitford 1991). Silence occurs when something becomes so natural that it does not need mentioning, or when an understanding loses out in the struggle to define the world, or alternatively, when something becomes so problematic that it cannot even be spoken about.

The object of investigation is the politico-administrative discourse that is understood both as a hegemonic discourse and as a field of competing discourses. The national politico-administrative discourse is the horizon that politicians, civil servants, experts and representatives of various interest groups apply when they speak and write about the social and political world. A discourse is a horizon that delimits the possible, what can be said and done, and the legitimate positions to be held (Dahl 2000; Norval 1996). The representatives of the state—the politicians and the civil servants—articulate an elite (expert) discourse. For Foucault, there are privileged discursive sites (Prado 1995), and the discourses stemming from these sites attain a particular authority related to their neutral, consensual style (Burton and Carlen 1979).

The original case study material consisted of all relevant commission reports, memorandums, internal reviews, laws and instructions covering the period 1996–2006.[2] The archive was established searching in various library databases as well as using snowball sampling to identify important texts that did not show up in the databases. Snowballing here refers to the inter-textuality occurring in between texts when one text refers to another. In a first round the total archive was read, identifying the major political problem and its solution. In this round, key texts that were particularly rich, ambiguous or represented ruptures were identified. Between two and eight key texts were identified for each year. In a second reading these key texts were analyzed more thoroughly with attention given to three analytical points of focus: governing, care and the identity of home helpers. Each text was analyzed according to the structures of recognition and misrecognition, as well as an attention to ambiguities in the texts indicative of struggles about understanding the social-political world. The purpose was to identify the dominant horizon(s) and rationalities (meaning), struggles in the texts (ambiguity) and absences (silences).[3] Quotations were selected that represent the richness of the material, relate to the analytical focus points and illustrate the results of the analysis.

A feminist discourse analysis implies attention to discursive effects (Bacchi 1999), such as the positions available in discourses and their potentially gendered character. Discursive effects are the effects that follow from the limits imposed on what can be thought and said by discourse (Bacchi 2009). Feminist discourse analysis also directs our attention to potentially gendering effects such as the ways discourses produce and transform gender and gendered subjectivities:

> Such an analysis would focus on the gendering of policy, institutions and organisations, and view gender*ing* as an incomplete and partial

process in which bodies and politics are always becoming meaningful. (Eveline and Bacchi 2005, 502)

To identify gendering in androgynous discourses, such as in the selected material, means identifying the framings of the home helpers, their work and qualifications. Gendering takes place both explicitly and implicitly through the way discourses regard and reward positions, that is, the way the position of home helpers, their work and qualifications are spoken of. The theory of recognition supports a critical evaluation of the gendered aspects of the discourse and the gendering positions, i.e., identifying the cultural valorizations at play. Leaving these methodological guidelines, I will now explain how Quality was created as the solution to a pile of problems in elderly care, and how the focus of NPM was redirected from efficiency to quality.

QUALITY—FROM STANDARDIZATION TO CONSUMERISM

In the mid nineties an attention to quality and ensuring the quality of services emerged as a primary concern for policy makers and top civil servants in Denmark.[4] The stress upon quality does not make efficiency as a key concern redundant, only less of a primary objective. In Danish reports such as *Handbook in User Involvement* (Socialministeriet 1997a) and *In Favour of a Freer Choice in Local Services* (Finansministeriet 1999), quality soon became the solution to the ills of elderly care such as an insufficient political control of the field, critical media coverage, the demographic development and what was seen as a new, more critical and demanding group of citizens.

The discourse about quality could be described as a two-tier track ensuring both 'the best and cheapest' services (Finansministeriet 2003; Højlund 2004). Three strategies were generally available in Danish NPM—these were a focus on quality, partnerships and contracts (Højlund 2004), and in elderly care, the strategy of quality became dominant. The Danish strategy of attention to quality involved both the application of standards of quality in the municipalities and increasing the choice of service users. This seeming paradox is related to the genesis of NPM as a dynamic marriage between two analytically different and partially contradictory logics, as mentioned previously. The different logics are, in Denmark, kept together by a dominant idea of change. In Denmark the logics of neo-liberal economics and managerialism have been translated into a specific institutional context resistant to retrenchment and outsourcing. The neo-liberal logic concentrates upon the introduction of markets and choice *and* the control of time, codification and the governance of details often characterized as Taylorism. The second logic of managerialism, inspired by Human Resource Management (HRM), stresses good leadership and development, applying concepts such as development, trust, dialogue, self-governance and self-governing groups (Dahl 2000; Greve 2003).

The neo-liberal logic has mostly been visible through the governing of details, which can be seen in the legislation about compulsory standards of quality. These quality standards at the level of municipalities outline the expected level of services generally and for various parts of care, as well as processes for ensuring the quality of services. The rationalities pushing for these standards are related to deeply embedded values of Weberian administration such as visibility and impartiality, and contrary to a social-democratic value of equality, making outsourcing highly controversial due to its presumed inequality. Due to resistance to outsourcing generally, and to outsourcing of elderly care more specifically, outsourcing was re-termed 'co-production' in Denmark. Co-production means dividing the production of care between private and public suppliers of home help based upon competition. This process necessitates that care provided in the private or state sphere be comparable. This in turn necessitates a codification of care, i.e., that the largely silent features of care be brought into language. This has happened primarily in the form of quality standards.

A good example of this way of thinking can be found in the publication *Standards of Quality: Examples of Best Practice* (Socialministeriet 2002). Standards of quality are believed to be useful governing tools providing more and better care for the same resources:

> If the municipality works consistently with governing and planning in elderly care a larger part of staff's time . . . can be used face-to-face with the elderly person. Therefore standards of quality are a useful tool. (51)[5]

Standards are believed to enable political control of the level of services and a more rational use of time. An interest in the governance of details is also prominent in the recommendation report *Model for the Specification of the Percentages of User Time in Elderly Care* (Socialministeriet 2004). The introduction of co-production (outsourcing) creates a need for the calculation of the consumption of time in public services. This calculation enables a comparison of prices with the private sector. The discourse specifies five categories of time use that are each specified at three levels. This is a comprehensive document containing a very detailed division of care into functions and a detailed form of governing, e.g., of direct user time. Direct user time is split into personal help, practical help and tasks outside the model such as nursing tasks. Personal help is again divided into personal care, mental care and care (*psykisk pleje og omsorg*), goal-oriented pedagogical tasks, treatments, nutrition, the giving of medicine, prevention and general health issues as well as various other kinds of help. These categories are again specified, e.g., various kinds of help that include help with transportation, help with the user's own administration (such as filling out forms, reading of letters from the municipality, help to administer their own money) and other activities such as contacting a GP, the hospital or other public authorities.

This new story of quality then, develops in two stages. In the first stage quality is believed to be reached by codifying care, that is, making it visible and measurable through the outlining of standards. Here the neo-liberal quest for competition creates a bureaucratic mastery of care by bringing it into speech—and a particular form of speech. In the second stage, quality becomes linked to the involvement of the user, since this involvement is in itself considered a quality through providing a voice for the elderly, giving more value for money (due to the targeting of services) and finally spurring the development of the professional (Socialministeriet 1997a). By 2003 quality in Denmark had developed a strong connection to consumerism where consumerism is understood as a belief that individual choice is an intrinsic good in itself (Glendinning 2008). In its second stage quality was linked more strongly to the second logic, that is, that inspired by human resource management (HRM). Elderly people increasingly become imagined as strong and self-determining, as freely choosing their own home helper and, more radically, acting as consumers choosing between public and private care. This logic is also being reproduced in the increasing attention to values as engineered by leadership. Value-based management is one of the main expressions of this logic in relation to the home helpers:

> The issue of chosen values is a key issue relating to the content of services and the performance of help. This is a key issue, since various concrete aims and results necessarily have to be related to the chosen values and their utilization in practice, if they are to be deemed useful. (Socialministeriet 2001, 58)

Despite their differences, the two logics co-exist in their simultaneous application in municipalities such as illustrated in the quotation below:

> In some of the chosen municipalities internal groups have been appointed in order to create a place for dialogue with the staff about free choice and the organizational changes implemented in the municipality. For the municipalities this has been a good investment. (Den sociale ankestyrelse 2003, 23)

Here HRM with a focus upon dialogue is combined with a neo-liberal focus upon the introduction of the market through a free choice. The HRM-inspired language of 'dialogue' here becomes a tool for ensuring the success of the neo-liberal logic.

The neo-liberal logic prevails throughout the period but with a shifting emphasis. In the beginning of the period standardization and an attention to details dominate, whereas in the end of the period limitations to this logic are clearly articulated. Increasingly, the discourse exposes the logic of self-governance for the elderly in relation to experiments with, amongst others, personal budgets (Rambøll Management 2006).

How does this change from quality as standardization to quality as consumerism happen? Needless to say, consumerism was part of the translation of NPM to Denmark early on, but it has gained prominence in recent years. Simultaneous with the increased stress on the choice of consumers, there is a continuous and increasing self-reflection in the discourse about the governance tools applied, including self-reflection about the suitability of standardization as a governing tool regulating the process of delivery. This self-reflection is most visible in a report written by the major stakeholders in the field in 2005 and in a feature article in one of the biggest Danish newspapers in 2007 written by key administrative experts.

In a major report entitled *Process Regulation of Counties and Municipalities* (Finansministeriet 2005), there occurs a meta-discursive reflection upon NPM standards such as ruling through a specification of process. This self-reflection upon the suitability of one of the logics of NPM does not threaten the dominance of NPM as such:

> [T]he municipalities, even though they are sceptical towards the amount of process regulation, do not want to abandon the regulation of processes. (2005, 77)

Instead, this self-reflection presents a crack in the horizon of understanding by outlining the limitations of one of the logics, such as the neo-liberal logic that is identified with the governance of details and standardization. One of the problems with this contemporary mode of governing is outlined in the discourses such as this:

> [T]he municipalities point out that one of the negative consequences of process regulation in elderly care is that the many formal demands have a tendency to redirect the attention of the employee from results towards the observance of rules in the process. (Finansministeriet 2005, 83).

Instead of focusing upon the client, the discourse articulates a problematic displacement towards the observance of rules and standards. Supporting this crack is an assertion of the autonomy of the municipalities in the report with words like *freedom of the municipality, the flexibility of the municipality* and their description of top down rules as a possessive system (*systemomklamring*). Self-reflection is also seen in the plea for forgiveness advocated by former leading civil servants in a feature article in a major Danish newspaper, *Politiken* (Hjortsdal et al. 2007). Please, forgive us, they argued. We did not know what we set in motion. They wanted governing through contracts, but instead of a new freedom, dialogue, increasing productivity and the quality of services, there was, in their view, an increase in the amount of bureaucracy. This mistake should, in their view, be corrected and there should be a return to the true NPM, such as leadership, development and the values of HRM. NPM had in their view, mistakenly stressed standardization and an all-encompassing governing of details.

New Public Management has entered a new phase in Denmark, stressing the quality of services. During the period from 1996–2006, quality was first framed as achievable through quality standards fusing the two logics of NPM and later on framed as identical with consumerism. During this period there was an increasing struggle about the proper understanding of NPM that attacked process-regulation and standardization as policy instruments that led to the production of red tape and goal displacement. This particular version of the neo-liberal logic has subsequently been weakened, leaving more space for HRM and other interpretations of the neo-liberal logic, such as a classic version of marketization.

STRUGGLES OVER CARE, GOVERNING AND IDENTITY

In describing institutions of recognition and misrecognition, as well as struggles over them, I have focused upon care, governing and identities. Care is rewritten in this period from co-responsibility (1997) to self-determination (2006). Care is also rewritten from personal help (1999) towards public services (2003). The radical ideal of self-determination is enabled by rewriting elderly people as empowered (Socialministeriet 1996, 47) and self-organizing (Socialministeriet 1997c, 23, 70). The ideal of capable and self-reliant elderly persons is not new. It was already present in the discourse up to 1996 (Dahl 2005b). The novelty is its radicalization, where care is no longer seen as a relationship developed reciprocally between the elderly person and his or her home helper, but rather a responsibilization of the elderly person. In the quotation below, this responsibilization can be seen with the image of an empowered and active elderly person:

> We know from experience that it is best for their energy, if they are in charge of their own activities. It can pacify the elderly if initiatives and decisions are issued by the municipality. The municipality should avoid embracing the activities of the elderly. (Socialministeriet 1996, 46)

Self-organizing is seen as improving the inner welfare of elderly persons (as set against the bogey of stigmatization), improving their sense of equality, normality and self-respect, and activities such as 'Elderly Helping Elderly' are emphasized as a model for self-organization and creating networks amongst the elderly (Socialministeriet 1997c, 23).

This ideal of self-determination, however, experiences resistance in the beginning of the period where the elderly are portrayed as more fragile and in need of safety, and as preferring a known, public provider:

[T]he impression that the majority of the elderly prefer a public provider that they know instead of a private enterprise they don't know
from experience. (Regeringen 2000)

This presents a major obstacle for the consumerist discourse that perceives
free choice as driven by the users and as creating more satisfaction amongst
the users (Regeringen 1999, 22–23). The problem voiced against free choice
is solved by introducing a limitation to free choice in the form of a division
between two kinds of elderly: the strong versus the fragile elderly person.
The strong elderly person is seen as capable of exercising a free choice, i.e.,
the self-determining elderly person taking up the responsibility of employer
in his/her own home (Rambøll Management 2006), whereas the fragile
elderly person lives in a nursing home. In the nursing home, dialogue and
the development of a common understanding amongst the elderly, relatives
and the staff is stressed as important:

> To increase the quality of care, it is important that all partners work
> together to find a common understanding of the limits and possibilities
> of a new life in a home for the elderly. This includes the elderly, their
> relative and the care persons. (Socialministeriet 2005, 11).

Simultaneously the ideal of governing changes from leadership focusing upon
targets (*målstyret ledelse*) (1997) to benchmarking (2002), standards of
quality (2004), evaluations (2004), self-evaluation (*egenkontrol*) (2004) and
reviews of user satisfaction (2004). There is a change from a relatively loose
form of governing to a more detailed form of governing both processes and
output. The texts reveal several struggles: one between the different levels
of the state involved in elderly care, and another struggle about the tools for
ensuring quality, which becomes pronounced towards the end of the period.

The first struggle is between the level of the nation state and the level of
municipality concerning the proper way of governing elderly care. This can
be seen in one of the important already-mentioned reports (Finansministeriet 2005) where the logic of process regulation (the neo-liberal logic) col-
lides with the logic of autonomy and flexibility (the logic of self-governance
and HRM):

> the top down state regulations of processes tend to become too specific
> and out of step with reality. (Finansministeriet 2005, 16)

Another struggle about governing is at the level of policy tools and is seen
in the three competing strategies concerning the best tool for ensuring
quality: that of dialogue, tests (for measurable qualifications) or the self-
determination of elderly (Socialministeriet 2005). Interestingly one voice is
missing. The elite discourse silences the home helper and their professional
knowledge as important in ideas about quality.

The identity of the home helper is radically rewritten from a weak, professional ideal to a relative silence concerning his/her identity. This silence was identified in the first round of reading where the professional changes from being spoken of to disappearing. The professional is in the beginning of the period imagined in a socio-pedagogical way with words such as prevention and activation and "having a solid knowledge of societal and health matters in a broad sense" (Socialministeriet 1996, 21). However, in 2005 the term 'home helper' disappears from the texts. The home helper is either silenced or very rarely described—and if so, described with words devoid of a professional component. S/he is named staff, supplier or performing staff. Very rarely is the terminology 'home helper' used. This new discourse of NPM functions along an older discourse of civil servants, i.e., like layering in the institutions (Thelen 2000).

In the beginning of the period there is a use of HRM words characteristic of the logic of self-governance. Words such as 'self-governing groups', 'groups' and 'dialogue' are applied in relation to the home helper. These disappear at the end of the period, indicating that HRM is being applied asymmetrically in the field and only directed at recipients of care. The performers of care, formerly seen as self-governing, disappear. HRM is framed within a more dominant logic of neo-liberalism, only giving space for the self-determination of recipients and not for home helpers.

NPM, RECOGNITION AND MISRECOGNITION

Do NPM and its two logics enable or restrain the recognition of home helpers? The analysis identifies both instances of recognition and misrecognition in the discourse where misrecognition refers to invisibility, lack of prestige and disrespect. Both institutions are illustrated, although most attention is paid towards the unjust institutions of misrecognition due to their prevalence in the analyzed understandings.

Generally speaking, NPM as a new story about elderly care implies new constructions of care that silence the professional element, positioning home helpers as suppliers and governing through a division between the governance of details and self-governance. The logics of neo-liberalism and of self-governance impact differently upon the recognition of home helpers. The neo-liberal logic produces, through the governance of details, a standardization that silences professional knowledge and assigns low status to home helpers and their specific knowledge of persons and processes acquired in the field. The home helper is rewritten as a manual worker doing practical work. Home helpers are increasingly invisible in the discourse, although they become less invisible as persons when elements of HRM are stressed. Their activities are only visible when inscribed in concepts such as 'functions' and 'services'.

The two logics produce together a focus upon quality that re-directs our attention towards the elderly as self-determining subjects, and sometimes even more radically as employers, and silences the home helper both as a person and as a professional. The home helper is seen as being at the disposal of the elderly person and as producing services, not care.

There are, however, aspects of NPM, such as HRM, that provide space for some recognition of home helpers and where the struggle between the two logics becomes apparent. A clear example of HRM as acknowledging the need for recognition is seen below in the quotation where the leader is referred to as 'she':

> She met a disappointed and frustrated staff in need of governance and support. They didn't feel recognised and didn't identify with the organisation. (Styrelsen for Social Service 2003, 46)

The need for being seen and heard is acknowledged and is, in this understanding, solved by introducing one of HRM's major concepts: 'good leadership'. Another aspect of HRM directs attention to the judgment and qualifications of home helpers such as seen in the quotation below:

> where the home helper in the situation decides whether it is defensible to replace a benefit. (Socialministeriet 2002, 18)

Here the home helper is granted autonomy, relying upon her qualifications to make a proper judgment. Qualifications in the logic of self-governance refer to personal qualifications such as judgment, motivation, flexibility and personal investment (Finansministeriet et al. 2002, 204). Qualifications cannot be seen as professional qualifications, which would collide too strongly with the dominant neo-liberal logic. They are, to a certain extent, being recognized as persons, but not as professionals.

This picture of a recognizing logic of self-governance, however, needs to be modified. The focus upon dialogue and communication in HRM seem to work against recognition of home helpers where problems of disrespect towards the home helpers become framed as problems of communication:

> Communication with the citizen is sometimes unsuccessful. It's necessary for the home helper to be aware of differences in clientele. In Ryvang twenty years ago it was normal to consider the home helper as a kind of maid, whereas the citizens in Kgs. Enghave would themselves have a background closer to the home helpers, wherefore problems of communication weren't as comprehensive. (Socialministeriet 2003a, 40)[6]

In this quotation, the discourse describes socio-historical reasons for problems of disrespect in a particular locality: Ryvang. These reasons relate to the different class positions of the elderly persons and the home helper and the tradition some time ago of having servants in upper middle class families such as those residing in Ryvang. The home helper is positioned as deficient and in need of improving her communication with the wording: "It's necessary for the home helper to be aware of differences in clientele." This frames disrespect as an individual problem of the home helper, i.e., a kind of responsibilization occurs where the problem is supposed to be solved by the home helper improving her/his communication. Problems of disrespect are individualized and re-inscribed into a discourse of self-governance such as in Human Resource Management. Here the state is passive towards instances of disrespect in treating home helpers as maids. The state does not grant them a reciprocal recognition, understood as in a position as social peers, but frames home helpers as co-responsible for the situation. The state affirms the difference of home helpers and does not actively attempt to change anachronistic patterns of social cultural valorizations amongst well-off elderly people.

Later on in the same text, the state notes the image problem of the home helpers (Socialministeriet 2003a, 57). However, the state remains silent on its own responsibility and does not outline strategies for changing this image problem.

Disrespect is also exposed in other texts describing home helpers as lazy and rigid (read: inflexible), indicating a more general institution of disrespect. A reference to their laziness can be seen here in a disparaging construction of home helpers where the Department of Social Affairs (Socialministeriet) uncritically quotes the head of one of the board of complaints:

> It is a risk that home helpers use the standard as a key, if they haven't a sufficient professional background or wrong attitude towards their work. That they, due to laziness, lean on the standard of quality. (Socialministeriet 2003b, 27)

Home helpers are described as leaning upon a pre-defined standard, suspending their active involvement and not being flexible. The inflexibility is a recurring issue since home helpers are produced as denying the performance of some services deemed outside their job:

> The employee sometimes exposes a rather rigid attitude towards the level of services. That causes a lot of dissatisfaction and complaints. (Socialministeriet 2003b, 26)

Flexibility is the ultimate goal, thereby silencing issues of health and safety at work, or lack of leadership as competing explanations. The discourse produces disrespect of home helpers by reproducing them on the wrong side of the dichotomy: flexibility versus rigidity.

The effects of NPM from a perspective of recognition demand an analysis of the two logics. This analysis shows that the neo-liberal logic quite unequivocally restrains the recognition of home helpers since it produces misrecognition either by silencing or imposing standards upon their work. The logic of self-governance, however, is quite ambiguous in its effects. On one hand, it acknowledges the need for recognition and granting autonomy to the home helpers. On the other hand, it reproduces disparaging constructions of them as inflexible and incapable of good communication, thereby reproducing disrespect twice, first by the elderly, and then secondly by a state only seeing a problem of communication, not of disrespect. Here a new mode of governing is illustrated with its strong individualization. Here structural problems of misrecognition are individualized onto the home helpers.

However, whether institutionalized misrecognition is reproduced at the level of municipalities as well depends crucially upon the translation processes between the administrative-politico discourse at the top level and that at the level of municipality. This is, however, the theme of another article (Dahl 2009).

CONCLUSION

The discursive context of home helpers changes with the rewriting of NPM from a preoccupation with efficiency to that of quality. Quality is, in the words of discourse theory, an empty signifier (Laclau 2002). This rewriting is joined by an increasing reflexivity about aims and available tools as well as change within NPM from a neo-liberal logic towards the logic of self-governance. The latter logic is applied asymmetrically in the horizon; only elderly people are supposed to be self-governing and self-determining, not home helpers.

Compared to the period prior to 1996, a radicalization of the self-determination of the elderly occurs along a binary view of the elderly as positioned in two groups: the strong and the weak. Whereas the strong elderly are visible and idealized as autonomous persons, the weak elderly seem to become marginal in the discourse. Here there is a parallel to the silencing of those who are fragile or helpless and conceived of as burdens that is taking place in the discourse advocated by the Disability People's Movement in the UK (Hughes et al. 2005). Both discourses draw upon a rationalized and male imaginary of independence and control, although the discourses originate from different sources. The discourse on self-determination by the Disability People's Movement is user driven, whereas the discourse on the self-determining elderly in the Danish politico-administrative discourse is engineered from above. What are the implications of this rewriting of the elderly? Whereas there is little doubt that self-determination works for disabled people (Hughes et al. 2005), I am less convinced that it works for elderly people *in toto*. Elderly people between these two poles of the binary face a difficult time being in-between categories, and there seems to be a disappearance of 'the unpleasant', understood as that which is fragile, helpless or burdensome.

Struggles over the ideals of care, identity and governing occur. Governing is split between a governance of detail (standards) and self-governance, wherein the home helpers are either silenced or standardized. Care is also rewritten from a relational model of co-responsibility to a one-way relationship with the elderly person as the employer and the home helper as staff or supplier. The state withdraws from a (weak) project of professionalization (Dahl 2000) to reproduce a strongly gendered, patriarchal state through the two logics. The neo-liberal logic framed as standardizations produce misrecognition of the home helper, rewriting her tasks from professional to non-professional ones. The other logic of human resources management—the logic of self-governance—is ambiguous, since on one hand it creates an attention to a home helper's personal qualifications, and on the other, rewrites disrespect as a problem of communication. The state individualizes the effects of a socio-cultural institution of disrespect by making this the problem of the home helper in question, and neither a political nor managerial problem.

This research was funded by the National Danish Research Council for the Social Science (Grant number 275–05–0226).

NOTES

1. The other dimensions of her theory of justice are redistribution and representation, which are not dealt with here. For an elaboration on these dimensions, please consult Fraser (2003, 2008).
2. I have identified the relevant material using search nouns like: home, home help, elderly care, service, care and social and health helpers in the databases.
3. The aim of my analytical strategy has not been an ambitious strategy of deconstruction, attempting to pull the system of identities and structures of recognition and misrecognition apart (Thompson 2006). Rather it has been a less ambitious attempt to identify discursive logics, the structures of recognition and misrecognition as well as to identify struggles about recognition.
4. A concern with quality took place earlier in one of the frontrunners of NPM, Britain, showing a less ideological, pragmatic attitude and with an increasing attention to what works (Ferlie et al. 1996; Newman 2001).
5. All translations from original Danish made by the author.
6. Ryvang used to be a residential area for the upper echelon of the middle class, as well as the upper class. Kgs. Enghave used to be an area where mainly skilled workers lived.

REFERENCES

Andersen, Niels Åkerstrøm. 2001. *Kærlighed og omstilling—Italesættelsen af den offentligt ansatte.* København: Nyt fra samfundsvidenskaberne.
Bacchi, Carol Lee. 1999. *Women, policy and politics.* London: Sage.

———— 2009. *Analysing policy: What's the problem represented to be?* Frenchs Forest: Pearson.

Bauman, Zygmunt. 2001. The great war of recognition. *Theory, Culture & Society* 18(2–3): 137–150.

Burton, Frank and Pat Carlen. 1979. *Official discourse.* London: Routledge and Kegan Paul.

Christensen, Tom and Per Lægreid. 2002. A transformative perspective on administrative reforms. In *New Public Management: The transformation of ideas and practice,* edited by Tom Christensen and Per Lægreid, 13–43. Aldershot UK: Ashgate.

———— 2007. Theoretical approach and research questions. In *Transcending New Public Management: The transformation of public sector reforms,* edited by Tom Christensen and Per Lægreid, 1–16. Aldershot UK: Ashgate.

Clarke, John and Janet Newman. 1997. *The managerial state.* London: Sage.

Dahl, Hanne Marlene. 2000. *Fra kitler til eget tøj—Diskurser om professionalisme, omsorg og køn.* Aarhus DK: Politica.

———— 2005a. Re-imagining the (welfare) professional as a specialized generalist. *Knowledge, Work & Society* 3(2): 19–39.

———— 2005b. A changing ideal of care in Denmark: A different form of retrenchment? In *Dilemmas of care in the Nordic welfare states: Continuity and change,* edited by Hanne Marlene Dahl and Tine Rask Eriksen, 47–61. Aldershot UK: Ashgate.

———— 2009. NPM, disciplining care and struggles about recognition. *Critical Social Policy* 29(4): 634–654.

Dean, Mitchell. 1999. *Governmentality: Power and rule in modern society.* London: Sage.

Den sociale ankestyrelse. 2003. *Frit valg på ældreområdet—15 kommuners erfaringer og brugernes oplevelser.* Copenhagen: Den sociale ankestyrelse.

Dunleavy, Patrick, Helen Margetts, Simon Baslow and Jane Tinkler. 2005. New Public Management is dead—long live digital-era governance. *Journal of Public Administration Research and Theory* 16(3): 467–494.

Eveline, Joan and Carol Bacchi. 2005. What are we mainstreaming when we are mainstreaming gender? *International Feminist Journal of Politics* 7(4): 496–512.

Feldman, L. C. 2002. Redistribution, recognition and the state. *Political Theory* 30(3): 410–440.

Ferlie, Ewan, Lynn Ashburner, Louise Fitzgerald and Andrew Pettigrew. 1996. *The New Public Management in action.* Oxford: Oxford University Press.

Finansministeriet. 1999. *Friere valg på de kommunale serviceområder.* Albertslund: Schultz Information.

———— 2003. *Fra få til mange leverandører.* Copenhagen: Finansministeriet.

———— 2005. *Procesregulering af amter og kommuner.* Albertslund: Schultz.

Finansministeriet et al. 2002. *Udfordringer og muligheder—den kommunale økonomi frem mod 2010.* Albertslund: Schultz Information.

Foucault, Michel. 1991. Governmentality. In *The Foucault effect: Studies in governmentality,* edited by Graham Burchell, Colin Gordon and Peter Miller, 87–104. Chicago: University of Chicago Press.

Fraser, Nancy. 1997. *Justice interruptus.* London: Routledge.

———— 2003. Social justice in the age of identity politics. In *Redistribution or recognition? A political-philosophical exchange,* edited by Nancy Fraser and Axel Honneth, 7–109. London: Verso.

———— 2008. *Scales of justice.* Cambridge: Polity Press.

Glendinning, Carole. 2008. Increasing choice and control for older and disabled people: a critical review of new developments in England. *Social Policy & Administration* 42(5): 451–469.

Greve, Carsten. 2003. *Offentlig ledelse—Teorier og temaer i et politologisk pers-pektiv.* Copenhagen: Jurist- og Økonomforbundets forlag.

Hansen, Hanne Foss. 2008. Forvaltningspolitiske reformer: kontinuitet eller brud? *Politik* 11(1): 6–17.

Hernes, Helga. 1987. *Welfare state and woman power: Essays in state feminism.* Oslo: Universitetsforlaget.

Hirdman, Yvonne. 1994. *Women: From possibility to problem? Gender conflict in the welfare state—The Swedish model.* Research Report Series no. 3. Stockholm: The Swedish Center for Working Life.

Hjortsdal, Henrik, Claus Nielsen, Jes Gjørup, Tommy Jensen, Leon Lerborg, Niels Refslund, Jakob Suppli og Jasper Steen Winkel. 2007. Tilgiv os—vi vidste ikke, hvad vi gjorde *Politiken*, March 29.

Hobson, Barbara. 2003. Recognition struggles in universalistic and gender distinctive frames: Sweden and Ireland. In *Recognition struggles and social movements*, edited by Barbara Hobson, 64–92. Cambridge: Cambridge University Press.

Højlund, Holger. 2004. *Markedets politiske fornuft.* Copenhagen: Samfundslitteratur.

Hood, Christopher. 1991. A public management for all seasons. *Public Administration* 69(1): 3–19.

Hood, Christopher and Guy Peters. 2004. The middle ageing of New Public Management: Into the age of paradox? *Journal of Public Administration Research and Theory* 14(3): 267–282.

Honneth, Axel. 1994. *Kampf um Anerkennung.* Frankfurt: Suhrkamp.

Hughes, Bill, Linda McKie, Debra Hopkins and Nick Watson. 2005. Love's labour lost? Feminism, the Disabled People's Movement and an ethic of care. *Sociology* 39(2): 259–275.

Johnson, Terry. 1995. Governmentality and the institutionalization of expertise. In *Health Professions and the State in Europe*, edited by Terry Johnson, 7–24. London: Routledge.

Knijn, Trudie and Stine Verhagen. 2003. Contested professionalism and the quality of home care. Paper presented at ESPAnet conference: Changing European Societies—The role for social policies, November 13–15, Copenhagen, Denmark.

Laclau, Ernesto and Chantal Mouffe. 1985. *Hegemony and socialist strategy.* London: Verso.

Laclau, Ernesto. 2002. Hvorfor betyder tomme udtryk noget i politik? In *Det radikale demokrati—Diskursteoriens politiske perspektiv*, edited by Ernesto Laclau and Chantal Mouffe, 135–146. Roskilde: Roskilde Universitetsforlag.

Larner, Wendy. 2000. Neo-liberalism: Policy, ideology and governmentality. *Studies in Political Economy* 63(3): 5–26.

Marcussen, Martin. 2002. *OECD og idespillet—Game Over?* Copenhagen: Hans Reitzels forlag.

Newman, Janet. 2001. *Modernising governance—New Labour, policy and society.* London: Sage.

Norval, Aletta. 1996. *Deconstructing apartheid discourse.* London: Verso.

Outshoorn, Joyce and Johanna Kantola. 2007. *Changing state feminism.* London: Palgrave.

Prado, C. G. 1995. *Starting with Foucault: An introduction to genealogy.* Boulder: Westview Press.

Rambøll Management. 2006. *Evaluering af Socialministeriets forsøg med personlige budgetter på hjemmehjælpsområdet.* Copenhagen: Slotsholmen.

Rausch, Dietmar. 2008. Diverging old-age care developments in Sweden and Denmark, 1980–2000. *Social Policy & Administration* 42(3): 267–287.

Regeringen. 1999. *Friere valg på de kommunale serviceområder.* Copenhagen: Schultz.

————. 2000. *Hvad sagde de? Høringer og borgerundersøgelse 2000*. Albertslund: Schultz.

Sahlin-Andersson, Kerstin. 2002. National, international and transnational constructions of New Public Management. In *New Public Management: The transformation of ideas and practice*, edited by T. Christensen and P. Lægreid, 43–73. Aldershot UK: Ashgate.

Schmidt, Vivien. 2002. Does discourse matter in the politics of welfare state adjustment? *Comparative Political Studies* 35(2): 168–193.

Socialministeriet. 1996. *Vejledning om sociale tilbud til ældre m.fl.*. Copenhagen.

————. 1997a. *Håndbog I brugerinddragelse—erfaringer fra socialministeriets kvalitetsprogram*. Copenhagen.

————. 1997b. *Styring af fremtidens hjemmepleje*. Ry: Socialministeriet.

————. 1997c. *Sociale Tendenser*. Copenhagen: PrePress.

————. 1998. *Vejledning om Lov om retssikkerhed og administration på det sociale område nr. 44 af 6.3*. Copenhagen.

————. 2001. *Kvalitetsstandarder I kommunerne*. Copenhagen: Socialministeriet 2002. *Kvalitetsstandarder I hjemmeplejen—eksempler på god praksis*. Odense: Syddansk universitetstrykkeri.

————. 2003a. *Evaluering af ældreserviceområdet—hvorfor kritik?* Evaluering. Copenhagen.

————. 2003b. *Ældrepolitiske forhold: Økonomi, ansvar og kritik. Sammenfatning af resultaterne fra Socialministeriets evalueringsprogram*. Copenhagen.

————. 2004. *Model til opgørelse af brugertidsprocenter (BTP) i ældreplejen*. Copenhagen: Socialministeriet.

————. 2005. *Hvad er kvalitet?* Copenhagen: Socialministeriet.

Styrelsen for Social Service. 2003. *Det der virker—10 historier om attraktive arbejdspladser i ældresektoren*. Odense: Glumsø bogtrykkeri.

Szebehely, Marta. 2003. Den nordiske hemtjänsten—bakgrund och omfattning. In *Hemhjälp i Norden*, edited by Marta Szebehely, 23–62. Lund: Studentlitteratur.

Taylor, Michael. 1994. The politics of recognition. In *Multiculturalism: Examining the politics of recognition*, edited by Amy Gutman, 25–73. Princeton: Princeton University Press.

Thelen, Kathleen. 2000. Timing and temporality in the analysis of institutional evolution and change. *Studies in American Political Development* 14(Spring): 101–108.

Thompson, Simon. 2006. *The political theory of recognition*. Cambridge: Polity.

Tully, Charles. 2000. Struggles over recognition and redistribution. *Constellations* 7(4): 469–482.

Vabø, Mia. 2006. Caring for people or caring for proxy consumers? *European Societies* 8(3): 403–422.

Verloo, Mieke and Emanuela Lombardo. 2007. Contested gender equality and policy variety in Europe: Introducing a critical frame analysis. In *Multiple meanings of gender equality*, edited by Mieke Verloo, 21–49. Budapest: Central European University Press.

Whitford, Margaret. 1991. *Luce Irigaray: Philosophy of the feminine*. London: Routledge.

Young, Iris Marion. 1990. *The Politics of difference*. Princeton: Princeton University Press.

8 Creating Home Care Recipients

Using Categorization as a Tool in Home Care Case Management

Anna Olaison

This chapter analyses the process of categorization in home care assessment meetings and case files. Older persons' requests for home care are dealt with through the processing of applications. The point of departure of this analysis is the idea that priorities are actively negotiated by the involved parties through interaction during assessment meetings and in the written documentation. The specific aim of this paper is to examine how welfare organizations such as those providing elderly care use categorization to deal with people's needs and how these practices have an impact on the decisions made. Looking for similarities as well as differences across cases, I explore the categorization process in two comparable situations—that is, situations in which the older persons are applying for similar services.

Although I consider home care assessments a locally negotiated social activity, assessments are also framed politically and institutionally. Home care assessments are framed politically by legislation in Sweden (i.e., the Social Welfare Act), and institutionally by the municipal policies and local guidelines concerning the types of home care services that can be provided. The care management process for home care in Sweden has many similarities with other European countries and has been the way that the provision of elderly care has been organized since the 1990s (Lindelöf and Rönnbäck 2004; Swedish National Board of Health and Welfare 2006a). The implementation of care management has also led to a more distinct focus on resource allocation which has resulted in more demands for documentation (Swedish National Board of Health and Welfare 2006b). Overarching this, the Swedish Social Welfare Act establishes a framework for the individual's rights; it interprets statutory obligations, formulating general guidelines at the local municipality level.

In Sweden home care assessments are usually made by municipal care managers[1] who meet with older people to form some idea of the need for help and discuss the steps to be taken. Swedish elderly care is characterized by a client-centered approach, where the law provides that the support must be furnished to the older person (Swedish Social Service Act (SFS) 2001, 453).[2] However during the last decade, home care in Sweden, as well as in the other Nordic countries, has become subject to resource constraints as well as to the introduction of a mangerialistic model of care management which has reduced the availability of home care services (Larsson and Szebehely 2006; Rauch 2007; Wrede et al. 2008). In combination with an ageing population, this has resulted in fewer people getting access to the formal service system, leaving the care to be provided by private and informal alternatives, often by relatives (Sand 2007; Stark 2007). Szebehely and Trydegård (2007) argue that the needs of older persons have not decreased and that the decline in publicly financed care services is more likely the result of the increasing difficulty of obtaining assessment-based assistance and a concomitant degradation in the quality and availability of care services. They assert that home care must be of a sufficient level of quality and comprehensiveness to appear as a feasible alternative for older persons. A view of older persons as active citizens with the ability to take advantage of what the market has to offer is emerging parallel to this trend toward an increasingly mangerialistic, market-based orientation.

Home care is subject to detailed regulation, and the focus of this chapter is the detailed assessment process through which the need for home care is established and, in particular, how processes of categorization are manifested in case files written by care managers. The frames of home care case management have to be translated and concretized with regard to the specific situation and person in question. This process of categorization is enacted as elderly persons and their needs for care are described in case files and they are transformed into home care recipients. This process is examined with focus on the ways written language is used as well as the mechanisms the language used brings into play. Studies of how elderly persons are processed through categorization and made into home care recipients may, thus, give an insight into how this process is handled in practice.

First, I give a brief introduction to research on documentation and categorization in social welfare work. This is followed by a description of methods and data used. A section then follows in which two case examples are used to illustrate the categories that take precedence in describing people's needs for home care.

DOCUMENTATION AND CATEGORIZATION

Documentation is integral to the practices of social welfare work, functioning as a tool organizations use to create and categorize clients (Hall, Slembrouck and Sarangi 2006; Spencer 1988).[3] Through categorizing, one transforms information about individuals, which then provides a basis for creating cases, i.e., something institutions can identify and work with. Then follows a process of handling the case through 'people processing', where the institution operates through a menu of pre-determined client categories (Prottas 1979: 4). In assessing home care applications, elderly persons' statements and wishes regarding home help are organized in case-file texts, formal documents that then represent decisions about services. This process of categorization creates the elderly person as home care recipient. In social work documentation, in fact, categories are used as resources for understanding, describing, explaining and making decisions about different kinds of support. It is the categorization of the specific case, or how a person is defined in relation to the institution's categories, that is crucial in determining what services are then available. Social workers within such activity systems, in turn, need to learn how to make sense of, and interact by means of, these materialized externalizations of human knowledge in order to handle their tasks and document their activities. These client categories are often based on category systems consisting of various administrative codes and classification systems that are used in organizing enterprises, and although these are often invisible to the public, they have a major impact on how reality is organized (Mäkitalo 2003; Smith 2001). As a result of an increasing focus on categorization, in order to construct clients, social work documentation has shifted towards the use of a more standardized evidence based language (White, Hall and Peckover 2008).

According to Hall (1997), categorization involves a process resulting in facts, opinions and events being established as one category succeeding another. Professional texts are also arranged in terms of story structures that are used as methods for negotiating the description of people and events and constructing versions for specific audiences (Hall 1997; Pithouse and Atkinson 1988). This means, for example, that describing an elderly person as needing care focuses on information emphasizing frailty in the person's medical and care condition.

Home care files are not merely vehicles of information; they also provide insight into the prevailing practice surrounding care of the elderly. Case-file texts are therefore not only rich in qualitative information about elderly care operations, but also articulate the reciprocal influence between care managers, bureaucracy and elderly persons constructed as home care recipients. According to Shotter (1993), categorization thus involves the institutional representative's making claims that render a specific category appropriate through a set of textual and verbal devices in order to legally establish that these claims are true; this, in turn, can demonstrate that this social worker can be held accountable for his or her work in relation to what is appropriate for the context. In home care, the defining of elderly persons' needs thus constitutes a foundation for categorization and functions as the tool care managers use to situate old people in relation to existing institutional resources.

The question of what *category of services* the elderly person belongs to is a specific version of a more general and central question about 'who the person is' and 'what kind of help' he or she needs. Rather than considering this as a matter of 'objective' diagnosis, I, in line with Hall, Slembrouck and Sarangi (2006), consider it as a matter of negotiating eventually competing versions of categorization.

Purpose and Questions

The overall purpose of this chapter is to show how categories are used in case-file texts in order to create older persons as home care recipients. The following questions are central: *How do care managers construct older persons as home care recipients in written documentation through case files? What categories have an impact for the decisions that are made?*

Methods

This case study comprises case files and decision documents in two home care cases. These documents constitute the main application for home care and were gathered as part of a larger research project in 2003–2004 in which the care management process was studied through assessment conversations, documentation and interviews (Olaison 2009). The case files included in this chapter came from two different social work districts in Sweden and the texts averaged 1½–2 pages.[4] In both cases, the elderly person applied for a security alarm and in both case files, the sought service had been approved, but the care management process and documentation were handled quite differently. One of the case-file texts also included pertinent case records in the form of running notes such as contacts, telephone conversations and measures taken. However, in this chapter I focus on the case-file texts, since these documents constitute the formal written public basis from which need for home care is specified and determined.

The case-file texts were studied using discourse analysis (Edwards and Potter 1996; Wetherell, Taylor and Yates 2003), a tradition focusing on how talk and text interact with, construct and comprise part of our lived reality. Accordingly, this approach aims at viewing the case-file texts as part of an ongoing discussion that surrounds the care of the elderly, the purpose of which is to shape images of, and to assess, elderly persons circumstances and needs for services. The case files were analyzed in terms of their sequential structure and contents and the categories used in presenting the elderly people and their needs.

The analysis was carried out in two steps. First, a close reading identified the structures of the case-file texts. Analysis indicated that there were differences in both the contents of the case files and in how the elderly person's needs were described and defined in them. After this, categories were identified for the different types of needs found, resulting in the identification of three main categories: medical, physical/care, and social needs.[5]

The following describes the written language used to present older people in two cases that both concerned home care but each handled the content differently. Excerpts from the assessments case-file texts identified as A and B are presented below as examples; all information about the elderly persons has been rendered anonymous and they have been given fictitious names.

COMPARING CASES: THE SAME SERVICE
BUT DIFFERENT DESCRIPTIONS

In both assessments cited below, the application concerned a security alarm; this is a relatively small and simple home care service but nonetheless is documented according to guidelines similar to those for other home care services. The case file texts had a tripartite structure made up of the initial report and decision sections. The texts were divided in a standardized way with similar headings, and give details and justify decisions about home care. The older persons in these cases had similar backgrounds: both were widows, around eighty years old and living alone in their own houses. Both wished to apply for a security alarm as both had fallen at home in the past and wished to be able to contact home care workers in the event of an accident. The assessments and case-file excerpts presented below are selected parts of texts in which the older person's social circumstances and state of health are presented. It was these passages that built up the case-file and conveyed an image of the older person's situation. The analysis concludes with examples concerning how the decisions and aims of the services are formulated.

The first case—case file A—concerns Mary, an 83-year-old woman who lives alone in a farm house. Mary is a widow and she suffers from Parkinson's disease, which has gradually decreased her mobility in both arm and legs. She now has difficulties moving her left arm and lifting her legs because of her tremors. As a result, she is now using a walker both indoors and outdoors for support. Her sons who live nearby are worried since Mary has fallen at home several times and has been unable to get in contact with her sons. This has had an impact on her everyday life as she is now afraid of going outside alone. Her sons want her to get some help with practical tasks such as cleaning and laundry as well as receive a security alarm. Mary wants to manage by herself but agrees to meet with the care manager to discuss the different options that can be provided by home care services. In the first excerpt below Mary's social circumstances are described.

The image conveyed of Mary's social circumstances is descriptive and objective. The information about her social network is limited to stating she has contact with friends; it does not describe the extent or nature of these relationships (example 1, lines 1–2). The reason for opening

---

Example 1. Excerpt from case file A regarding social circumstances

Mary lives in a farmhouse. Her husband died in Dec. 2000. Has good contact with old school friends. Mary, who has Parkinson's, has fallen several times, but has then been able to get up on her own. [She] is now a bit worried that something might happen to her and [she will] then not be able to contact anyone. Mary also feels a bit worried that some unauthorized person could get in and is applying for a security alarm so as to be able to call for help in emergencies. Otherwise, Mary manages with some help from her sons.

the case file is described: Mrs. X has Parkinson's disease and has fallen several times (line 3). When the need is to be justified, a descriptive subjective argument is used, based on the older person's experience of her circumstances as insecure: "[she] is now a bit worried that something might happen [to her]" (line 4). The next sentence describes her fear that "some unauthorized person could get in" (lines 5–6), but no further information is given about what caused this fear; rather, the fear is cited to strengthen and develop the case file concerning why a security alarm would be a legitimate service. The report about Mary's social circumstances concludes with a factual statement about her functions and her relationships with her closest relatives, her sons (lines 7–8). The text is clear that she receives help from her children, but the extent and nature of the help is not indicated; it is simply recorded in the case file and is not mentioned further. This can be interpreted as indicating that this factor has no bearing on the decision to grant an alarm or that relatives' contributions have little significance for the assessment.

The second case file, presented below, concerns another application for home care which ends up with the same service, a security alarm. This case—case file B—concerns Anne, who is an 84-year-old widow who lives alone in a house in a middle-sized municipality. Anne has two sons who live in other parts of the country and who are unable to help her with daily practical tasks. The older person's social circumstances are also described under the heading "social circumstances and residence." Anne's health has been getting worse, especially her eyesight, and both Anne and her sons are worried that she will not be able to manage to maintain living in the house much longer. Anne is also anxious about her security, living alone and with the possibilities of falling. Below Anne's social circumstances are described in the case file.

Example 2. Excerpt from case file B regarding social circumstances

Anne said she was born in [country x] and moved to Sweden at the end of the 1940s. She has lived alone since her husband's death in 1993, in a villa with four rooms, kitchen, and cellar. Anne said she has so far managed the cellar stairs. There are also stairs to the ground level to the outer door. Anne said further that she has three sons, Philip, John, and Oscar; none lives in the city, but she has regular contact with and visits from them. Anne feels lonely and abandoned. She has found it hard to find friends who have the same interests as she does. Anne feels great anxiety about maintaining the house, which she no longer has strength for. She says she has thoughts of moving into a flat, but worries about how that would go, purely practically, but also whether she would feel at home anywhere else.

This case file gives biographical background about an older woman (example 2, lines 1–2). It also provides objective descriptive mapping of her social network, her contact with her sons and the layout of her home (lines 2–5). What characterizes this case file is that it includes direct quotations from the older woman from the dialogue that took place during the assessment conversation. This is done for example, by indicating "Anne said she has so far managed" (line 3) or "Anne said further" (line 5). In this type of case file, the argument concerning the older person's social circumstances is built more on subjective feelings such as "Anne feels lonely and abandoned" (line 7) and "feels great anxiety about maintaining the house" (lines 8–9). We are also acquainted with other matters that do not directly pertain to the case file's actual purpose, applying for an alarm, but to the subject's thoughts about moving house (lines 10–12). This peripheral detail strengthens the narrative and more clearly elucidates the woman's situation concerning her sense of insecurity and anxiety; it is not, however, followed up later in the case-file text.

In the next part in the case-file texts, the report section touches on the older person's state of health described in case file A as follows:

Example 3. Excerpt from case file A regarding state of health

Parkinson's for about five years uses crutches to walk. Otherwise healthy.

Here Mary's state of health is described with an objective statement about her condition and how long she has had Parkinson's (example 3, line 1). There is no information about the consequences of the disease or how it affects the woman's daily life; instead, the same sentence focuses on the aids she uses for getting about in her home. The passage ends with the statement "Otherwise healthy," which can be interpreted as an objective summary of the care manager's assessment of the woman's general health.

In case file B, Anne's state of health is described in more detail:

Example 4. Excerpt from case file B regarding state of health

Anne reported that two days ago she had to go to emergency as she had pain in the right eye. The doctor stated from the cranial X-ray that she had a thrombus in the back part of her brain. She is taking anti-coagulant medicine. Anne said that she is seeing worse, her eyes feel tired, and her balance is impaired. [Sixteen words cut] Anne reported that she feels as if there is crawling inside her muscles, especially on nights when she has trouble sleeping. She said she is also troubled by sweating, which she sees as psychologically conditioned. Anne takes tranquilizing medication. Anne said otherwise that she manages her daily life without major problems.

Examples 3 and 4 convey a largely similar image of the two women's state of health: they both have health problems from failing functions and various illnesses but despite this are managing their everyday lives. However, the description is significantly more thorough in case file B, where a thrombus in the brain and, in relation to this, a hospital stay, are documented in detail from the woman's subjective experience of the event and her state of health since (example 4, lines 1–5). Unlike case file A, case file B also reports statements from other professionals, here the doctor's statement about her medical condition (lines 2–3). Furthermore, the older person's subjective experiences of her state of health were reported by the care manager's rendering the narrative through reported speech: *Anne reported* and *Anne said that* (lines 4, 5, and 9). There is also a hint of the woman's possibly having psychological problems from her own testimony about sweating, but it is not followed up further in the case-file text (line 8). Here, too, the passage describing state of health concludes by reporting the woman's subjective statement that despite her health troubles she is managing well (lines 9–10). This information may be used by the care manager to help justify the later decision 'only' to grant a security alarm.

When it comes to the decision section of the case file, the assessment and aim are justified by the decision under the assessment/goal heading:

Example 5. Excerpt from case file A regarding assessment/goal

Mary, who has Parkinson's and has fallen on several occasions, is applying for a security alarm. To enable her to call for help in emergency situations due to functional disability, it is recommended that a security alarm is granted. By granting Mary a security alarm she can live securely and independently and obtain a reasonable quality of life.

The basis for assessment is an objective description in which facts from previous sections are repeated. The reason for granting assistance is explained through an argument that builds on possibilities and the need to be able to summon help in emergencies (example 5, lines 1–3). Functional disabilities are also cited as a reason for the grant. Furthermore, it is indicated that the goals of the service are that the woman should feel secure and be able to live independently (lines 4–5); these goals are wholly in line with the guidelines set forth in the Swedish Code of Statutes (SFS 2001, 453) that older people should be guaranteed a certain standard of living.

The assessment passage and decision section in case file B is characterized by the professional's perspective and the personal assessment is brought out more clearly than in case file A.

> **Example 6. Excerpt from case file B regarding assessment/goal**
>
> *The undersigned assesses that Anne needs the sought service as she lacks proximity to relatives, but also due to the anxiety she has experienced since the thrombus and at not managing home maintenance, along with the prospect of making a decision to move house. A security alarm will allow Anne to contact home care staff round the clock if she should need help with something she cannot manage on her own. Through this service Anne is deemed able to attain a reasonable standard of living.*

In example 6 we see how the care manager explicitly states that she is making an assessment. What justifies the decision is chiefly the woman's lack of support in the form of a close social network and that she feels anxiety and insecurity (example 6, lines 1–4). The function of the security alarm in the woman's everyday life is also justified here by stating that the ability to contact support staff day and night itself constitutes security (lines 5–7). Here, too, standardized formulations concerning what constitutes a reasonable standard of living are stated later in the assessment to establish the decision in relation to the legislation (lines 7–8). However, the formulation of aims in case file B is imbued more with the older person's perspective on a personal level, i.e., what it might mean practically, and emphasizes more positive aspects as well, for instance that help in the home can help in maintaining independence and autonomy in everyday life (lines 7–8).

As noted above, there were marked differences between case files A and B in how the need for a security alarm was documented. The case files showed variety in both content and level of detail used to describe the life circumstances and events leading to the decision to grant a security alarm. Although the case files were structured in similar ways, using a fixed frame of headings, the care managers used different language to describe the older person's needs. In case file A more facts, based on medical and physical categories, were used as compared to case file B. Case file B reflected more of the interactional dynamics from the assessment conversation, and the elderly person's own storyline was more visible. Similar differences were also found in case-file texts in another study with a broader sample (Olaison 2010) where two basic types of case-file texts, the event oriented and the more fact based, were found. Case files that had a fact-oriented style tend to rely more on medical categories and event-oriented case files took more account of social circumstances.

Previous studies have further shown that case files use social categories mostly for describing the living circumstances and social networks of the clients. They have in fact little impact on decisions (Olaison forthcoming; White, Hall and Peckover 2008). This case analysis shows, in line with this, that medical and physical categories were superior to the social arguments in decision making. Case files are also usually written for organizational purposes, where categories are used for locating the clients within the institutional frames (Prottas 1979). As home care practice becomes subject to far-reaching cost restraints, it is not surprising that priorities are established that stress medical and physical needs. Granting a security alarm can be seen as a relatively small home care service. The decision to provide this service can be seen as a preventive measure, making the elderly persons feel secure and able to live independently at home for as long as possible. Nevertheless, the process of getting access to this small service included the documentation of several personal details, a process that did not differ much from the information gathered in cases handling a greater amount of home care services (Olaison 2010). This poses important issues related to the applicants' personal integrity, as well as questions concerning the relevance of the magnitude of information needed for granting a security alarm. Also, the life view or wishes of the elderly applicants are hardly reflected upon in the case files. If their perspective is present in the text (as in case file B), it is most often used to present events leading up to the present situation or to get a picture of the person's social network. Therefore it may be said that the documentation does not reflect the person-centered holistic approach that is advocated in the Swedish code of statues, but instead are based more on abstract categories such as a particular isolated services.

Concluding Comments

Home care in many European countries has undergone an extensive restructuring and is constantly changing in terms of both its organization and the conditions under which care can be provided (Fine 2007; Postle and Beresford 2007; Wrede et al. 2008). As a result of this development, documentation has shifted towards a more standardized, evidence-based language (Taylor 2008; White, Hall and Peckover 2008). Previous research has shown that local policies and guidelines govern the home care assessment process, creating dilemmas for care managers' assessments (Ceci 2006; Janlöv 2006; Postle 2002). This has resulted in more standardized processes and fewer possibilities of providing care outside the standardized catalogue with the consequence that relevant needs may be neglected (Petersson and Smitdt 2003).

Categorization plays a significant role in institutional welfare settings and functions as a tool for sense making and co-ordination of perspectives and activities (Mäkitalo 2003). Welfare workers use categories to contextualize and define clients (Cedersund and Olaison 2010; Hall, Slembrouck and Sarangi 2006; Mäkitalo 2006). However, case files tend to ignore the interactional dynamics, not reflecting all the particulars that can exist in a case discussion (Hall, Slembrouck and Sarangi 2006; Olaison 2009). The case analysis conducted in this chapter shows no exception from this, even though the care managers use categories in different ways to construct elderly persons as clients. Medical and physical categories were given precedence over social categories in the decision section in both cases and were used to construct the elderly persons as suitable clients for receiving a security alarm. This indicates, in line with other studies, that the home care case files are controlled by a fixed organizational frame in the striving for standardization (Olaison 2010). A holistic life view should, according to present legislation, be applied. Present findings suggest that such a view may be lost by the impact of a mangerialistic new public management thinking.

In their present status, home care case-files harbor an inherent dilemma. The documentation needs to be developed further on several levels to support clients and families, while at the same time protecting individual rights. Although this chapter builds on a small case analysis, it highlights the importance the categorization process has for the outcome of decisions. Categories used in social services are often embedded in routines for maintaining institutional order (Hall, Slembrouck and Sarangi 2006; Juhila et al. 2003; Lipsky 1980), often in relation to predetermined systems and administrative codes, and importantly, often are invisible to the public. They have, however, a major impact on how practice is organized (Mäkitalo 2006). Further studies looking more closely at particular acts of social action in the field of home care practice are warranted. By studying these practices on a micro level we can access how and in what ways the discourse surrounding welfare services is implemented.

NOTES

1. Municipal care managers are often trained social workers and during assessment meetings help of both physical and practical kinds are usually discussed.
2. Assessments of older persons' assistance should, according to the Swedish National Board of Health and Welfare (2006a), be guided by a holistic approach in which such needs are viewed as subjective, personal and variable.
3. The theoretical part on categorization above has previously been published (see Olaison 2010). Permission to publish a modified version has been given by SAGE Publishing.
4. Quoted documents were translated by the author from Swedish to English and then edited by a translation firm.
5. Physical needs include needs for practical help and care help in relation to functional impairments. Social needs include charting the older person's networks, activities and available informal services and other needs of a social and existential nature. Medical needs include various diagnoses of ill health and cognitive difficulties.

REFERENCES

Ceci, Christine. 2006. "What she says she needs doesn't make a lot of sense": practices of seeing in home care case management. *Nursing Philosophy* 7: 90–99.

Cedersund, Elisabet and Anna Olaison. 2010. Care management in practice: on the use of talk and text in gerontological social work practices. *International Journal of Social Welfare* 19: 339–347.

Edwards, Derek and Jonathan Potter. 1996. *Discursive psychology.* London: Sage.

Fine, Michael. 2007. *A caring society? Care and the dilemmas of human service in the twenty- first century.* New York: Palgrave Macmillan.

Hall, Chris. 1997. *Social work as a narrative.* Aldershot UK: Ashgate.

Hall, Chris, Stefan Slembrouck and Srikant Sarangi. 2006. *Language practices in social work. Categorisation and accountability in child welfare.* London: Routledge.

Janlöv, Ann-Catrine. 2006. Participation in needs assessments of older people prior to public home help. PhD diss., Lund University, Sweden.

Juhila, Kirsi, Tarja Pösö, Chris Hall and Nigel Parton. 2003. Introduction: Beyond a universal client. In *Constructing clienthood in social work and human services: Interaction, identities and practices,* edited by Chris Hall, Kirsi Juhila, Nigel Parton and Tarja Pösö, 11–26. London: Jessica Kingsley Publishers.

Larsson, Kristina and Marta Szebehely. 2006. Äldreomsorgens förändringar under de senaste decennierna. [Changes in care of the elderly in recent decades]. In *Äldres levnadsförhållanden. Arbete, ekonomi, hälsa och sociala nätverk 1989–2003,* edited by Joakim Vogel, 411–420. Stockholm: SCB.

Lindelöf, Margareta and Eva Rönnbäck. 2004. *Att fördela bistånd: Om handläggningsprocessen i äldreomsorgen.* [Distributing assistance to the elderly: The case handling process in elder care]. PhD diss., University of Umeå Sweden.

Lipsky, Michael. 1980. *Street-level bureaucracy. Dilemmas of the individual in public services.* New York: Russell Sage Foundation.

Mäkitalo, Åsa. 2003. Accounting practices as situated knowing: dilemmas and dynamics in institutional categorization. *Discourse Studies* 5: 495–516.

———. 2006. Arbetslöshet och institutionell kategorisering. In *Att hantera arbetslöshet: Om social kategorisering och identitetsformering i det senmoderna.* [Handling unemployment: On social categorization and identity formation in late modernity], edited by Åsa Mäkitalo, 43–66. Stockholm: Arbetslivsinstitutet.

Olaison, Anna. 2009. Negotating needs. Processing older persons as home care recipients in gerontological social work practices. PhD diss., University of Linköping Sweden.

——— 2010. Creating images of old people as home-care receivers: categorizing needs in social work case files. *Qualitative Social Work* 9: 500–518.

——— (forthcoming). Requests and outcomes in care management. Processing older persons as client's thorough talk and text in old age care. *Journal of Social Work.*

Petersson, L. and M. Smitdt. 2003. *Prosjekt faelles sprog: Et forsøg på styrning genem ensretning i hemmehjelpen.* [Project common language: An attempt for governance through standardization in home-based care]. Copenhagen: Akademiskt forlag.

Pithouse, Andrew and Paul Atkinson. 1988. Telling the case: Occupational narrative in a social work office. In *Styles of Discourse,* edited by Nicholas Coupland. Beckenham: Croom Helm.

Postle, Karen. 2002. Working between the idea and the reality: ambiguities and tensions in care managers' work. *British Journal of Social Work* 32: 335–351.

Postle, Karen and Peter Beresford. 2007. Capacity building and the reconception of political participation: a role for social care workers? *British Journal of Social Work* 37(1): 143–158.

Prottas, Jeffery M. (1979). *People processing. The street level bureaucrat in public services bureaucracies.* Lexington: Lexington Books.

Rauch, Dietmar. 2007. Is there really a Scandinavian social service model? a comparison between childcare and elderly care in six European countries. *Acta Sociologica* 50: 249–269.

Sand, Ann-Britt. 2007. The value of the work—on employment for family care in Sweden. In *Family caregiving for older and disabled people*, edited by Isabella Paoletti, 295–319. New York: Nova Publishers.

SFS. 2001. *The Swedish code of statutes Social Service Act*. Stockholm: The Swedish Parliament.

Shotter, John. 1993. *Conversational realities. Constructing life through language*. London: Sage.

Smith, Dorothy E. 2001. Text and the ontology of organisations and institutions. *Studies in Cultures, Organization and Society* 7: 159–198.

Spencer, William J. 1988. The role of texts in the processing of people in organizations. *Discourse Processes* 11: 61–78.

Stark, Agneta. 2007. Warm hands in cold age—on the need for a new world order of care. In *Warm hands in cold age*, edited by Nancy Folbre, Lois Shaw and Agneta Stark, 7–18. London: Routledge.

Swedish National Board of Health and Welfare. 2006a. *Socialt arbete med äldre. Förslag till kompetensbeskrivning för handläggare inom äldreomsorg*. [Social work with old people: Recommendations for a description of qualifications for care managers in old-age care]. Stockholm: Socialstyrelsen.

——— 2006b. *Vård och omsorg om äldre- lägesrapport 2005*. [Old age care, 2005]. Stockholm: Socialstyrelsen.

Szebehely, Marta and Gun-Britt Trydegård. 2007. Omsorgstjänster för äldre och funktionshindrade: Skilda villkor, skilda trender? [Care services for old and disabled persons: Different requirements, different trends?] *Socialvetenskaplig tidskrift* 14: 197–219.

Taylor, Carolyn. 2008. Trafficking in facts: writing practices in social work. *Qualitative Social Work* 7: 25–42.

Wetherell, Margret, Stephanie Taylor and Simeon Yates. 2003. *Discourse theory and practice*. London: Sage.

White, Sue, Chris Hall and Sue Peckover. 2008. The descriptive tyranny of the common assessment framework: technologies of categorization and professional practice in child welfare. *British Journal of Social Work* 38: 1–21.

Wrede, Sirpa, Lea Henriksson, Håkon Høst, Stina Johansson and Betina Dybbroe. 2008. Care work and the competing rationalities of public policy. In *Care work in crisis*, edited by Sirpa Wrede, Lea Henriksson, Håkon Høst, Stina Johansson and Betina Dybbroe, 15–33. Lund: Studentlitteratur.

9   The Making of Medico-Managerial Care Work Culture in Public Home Care for the Elderly[1]

Lea Henriksson and Sirpa Wrede

Municipal home care for the elderly provides a good example of the recent welfare policy shift in Finland and its implications for care work cultures and professional agency. Since the 1990s, the scope of public services aimed at the elderly has been narrowed down through policies formulated under the influence of neo-liberal ideologies and the deepest recession in the Finnish economy since the 1930s. The restructuring of public sector services has been aimed at breaking down institutional care and limiting elderly care to the so-called basic services and reallocating these services to the frailest elderly (Julkunen 2001; Paasivaara 2002; Wrede and Henriksson 2005). The logic guiding the narrowing down of the public services is economic and technocratic. That is, the production of public services now relies on a logic of cost-effectiveness as well as medical and managerial criteria and expertise.

Since the early 1970s different groups of professionals working in or contributing to public home care, including primary health center doctors, have been employed by municipalities (Henriksson and Wrede 2004). Until the 1980s, state regulation underpinned the democratization of professionalism and supported the agency of frontline care workers, both in terms of their employment rights and their control over their work (Henriksson, Wrede and Burau 2006). When the institutional matrix of elderly care in the welfare-mix era was demarcated, the expertise of socially defined care was devalued and excluded and the agency of care workers started to disintegrate (Wrede and Henriksson 2004).

The exclusion of socially defined care from municipal home care for the elderly in Finland[2] is here recognized as a crisis in terms of the erosion of the skills and competence of frontline care workers. Instead of valuing the expertise of socially defined care, the reorganization limited the frontline care workers' scope for self-steered work, and their mandate was increasingly defined through the expertise of others, primarily managers, doctors or nurses. Parallel to these changes, the terms and conditions of the turbulent public sector labor market created unsafe employment conditions. Here the rapid ageing of the Finnish population is expected to present an overwhelming workload for the welfare state that is worsened by the impending shortage of labor in care work.

This chapter examines the institutional matrix of public care services. By 'institutional matrix' we refer to the institutions—the organizations, rules, routines, procedures and assumptions—that shape the public care services and the division of labor in care work (Freeman 1999, 91). We consider how the changes referred to above have reframed the care work culture and redefined the frontline care workers' agency. By 'care work culture' we refer to the welfare state ethos underpinning the services—that is, the kinds of services provided, who is eligible to receive them and the kinds of skills and competence the provision of these services require.

In the following, we first consider institutional shifts in the development of municipal home care for the elderly[3] paying particular attention to how the universalist welfare state reformed the Finnish care work culture and the position of frontline carers. The second section examines the impact of neoliberal policy reforms at the national-level on the scope of public elderly-home care. The third section draws attention to the implementation of these reforms, from the perspective of the meso-level of the municipality, of which the City of Helsinki is used as an example. Furthermore, we highlight the collective agency of care workers and consider how the trade unions representing the different groups of care workers—public health nurses, nurses, practical nurses—with a stake in public elderly home care have responded to the reforms. In the conclusion we consider the described changes in the institutional matrix as a dynamic process that has impoverished the care work culture in public elderly home care in Finland. It has removed the mandate for care workers to provide comprehensive socially defined care. Instead, public elderly home care now only entails services that are defined as 'basic'.

THE RISE OF SOCIALLY DEFINED CARE: FROM HOME HELP TO HOME CARE

Before the 1960s, it was difficult to talk about an elderly care system or even formal occupations in the provision of care to the Finnish elderly. The situation changed when public home help services specifically directed to the elderly were created in 1966 through the Municipal Home Help Act (Simonen 1990). The new service offered assistance in daily routines, enabling the elderly to continue living in their homes as long as possible. At the same time, home help services created a basis for the gradual formalization of occupations that provided socially defined care.

The Municipal Home Help Act was a sign of a new way of thinking in response to the pressures caused by urbanization and women's increased involvement in the labor market. In cultural terms, the home helpers represented a traditional view of how care for the elderly was to be organized. Home help workers were typically former housewives who had a short training course on housekeeping tasks. Thus their formal qualifications were strikingly modest if compared with more regulated health care occupations (Rauhala 1996). The occupation was eventually shaped by the policy into a *homemaking culture* (cf. Waerness 1992), in which the home helpers occupied what could be identified as a boundary role in the municipal administration. The homemaking service provided by the helpers enabled the elderly to continue their everyday lives largely in the way to which they were accustomed, without becoming dependent on relatives or friends (Simonen 1990; Tedre 1999; Waerness 1984). Some clients held onto traditional ideas of private service, trying to treat helpers as 'municipal maids'. However, the legislation underpinning the institutional position of the municipal home helpers as public service employees provided them protection from this attitude by making them, first and foremost, responsible to the municipality (Tedre 1999, 2004).

In the 1980s, policy makers and researchers sought to academize socially defined care as a specific expertise in 'social care'. The new expertise was supported by a knowledge base deriving from social gerontology (Koskinen et al. 1988; Paasivaara 2002; Tedre 1999). While the traditional home-help service emphasized household chores such as cleaning, cooking and shopping, the new social care treated these tasks as secondary. In the social care perspective, instead of caring for the home, the focus was to be on interaction and the needs of the elderly person (Borgman 1998, Tedre 1999). Many scholars have criticized this reformulation of the knowledge base as underpinning a professionalist hierarchy of so-called dirty work (e.g., Tedre 2004). On the positive side, however, the redefinition of home help as social care was part of the rise of elderly care as a policy frame. In this framework the elderly person was recognized as a citizen, entitled to care in his or her own right. Elderly care policy promoted individualism and humanism as the ideals that were to form the core of the ethos of elderly care. This was the foundation for the reframing of home help into home care (Paasivaara 2002). Thus the scientific formulation of the knowledge base was part and parcel of the professional projects of the universalistic welfare state (Julkunen 1994). From the point of view of care workers, the state support for professionalizing socially defined care also contributed to more egalitarian working conditions and employment safety (Henriksson and Wrede 2004; Henriksson, Wrede and Burau 2006).

In 1988, 46.2% of the Finnish population aged 75 or older received home help services. Of these, 17.6% received long-term residential care of some type (Vaarama and Noro 2005). Reflecting the expansion of elderly home help in the 1980s, the number of care workers in home care service increased to approximately 13,000 people (Vaarama et al. 2001). This group was one of the largest in the care sector and most care workers worked full-time. Even though the home care personnel consisted of almost equal shares of the lower-grade home helpers and the higher-grade homemakers, their work roles and positions as public sector employees had become increasingly similar (Rauhala 1996; Simonen 1990).

The institutional matrix of the welfare state expansion era made public services readily available on the basis of broadly defined needs. At the same time, however, the figures reflect the long-term Finnish tradition of investing in institutional care rather than in ambulatory services. Elderly home care and residential housing services for the elderly remained only secondary in elderly care policy despite their positive connotations as more 'humane' forms of care (Paasivaara 2002). Thus despite the efforts to develop the knowledge base of municipal home help, the most valued forms of expertise remained associated with institutional care. Furthermore, when compared with other forms of socially defined care, particularly child day care, Finnish elderly home care was always based on weak universalism that in recent years has eroded (Kröger, Anttonen and Sipilä 2003). Although the public responsibility for elderly care is still extensive, the expectation is that the informal networks will complement the formal service.

NEO-LIBERAL POLICIES BOOSTING THE MEDICAL CULTURE IN ELDERLY HOME CARE

The institutional restructuring of the Finnish welfare state in the direction dictated by the neo-liberal ideology kicked off in the early 1990s with the decentralization of the responsibility for welfare budgets and planning and organizing welfare services to the autonomous municipalities.[4] The new welfare-mix matrix, implemented through legislation in 1993, encouraged municipalities to purchase health and social services from other service providers rather than providing them directly. The reorganization of service production was accompanied by education policy aiming at shaping a flexible workforce for the diverse settings of service provision.

Four important ideological starting points directed the neo-liberal reforms of Finnish elderly home care. Firstly, the care provided by a family member was defined as the favored solution in elderly care. Accordingly, from the year 1988 to the year 2002, the volume of family care assistance increased by 49% (Vaarama and Noro 2005). Secondly, the idea of a welfare mix was to be implemented with the aim of achieving cost-efficiency for the municipality and availability of choice for the elderly. Reflecting this idea, the role of the public sector was to a large extent reorganized corresponding to the so-called purchaser-provider model (Kovalainen 2004; Vaarama and Noro 2005).

Thirdly, in search of efficiency in the use of municipal resources, national policy makers promoted trans-sectoral home care services, merging socially defined care with medical care, as the favored solution to the challenge of dismantling institutional care. Home nursing was assigned the central role in making home care capable of managing clients who would previously have been cared for in institutions. Furthermore, instead of recognizing comprehensive responsibility, the role of the public sector was restricted to producing 'basic services' that were ideally provided through a welfare mix. Our earlier study indicates that policy makers privileged medical needs when defining which services were recognized as 'basic' (Wrede and Henriksson 2004). Accordingly, the reframed elderly home care was underpinned by an ethos that Waerness (1992) defines as *professional medical culture.*

The fourth starting point for the neoliberal reforms in home care was promoting the deinstitutionalization of care. Home care was assumed to combine the goals of providing both more affordable as well as a more humane and client-centered form of elderly care than institutional care. However, contrary to the goal of developing home care into a well-built service that readily replaces other more expensive forms of care, municipalities did not, in the 1990s, generally invest in this service. Instead many municipalities shifted resources from both municipal home care and residential homes to service housing (Vaarama and Noro 2005). The establishment of service housing units was expedited through state sponsorship and great ideological expectations were directed toward this service. Service housing was to provide a choice for the client, thus promoting the emphasis on service quality. However under the severe financial pressures of the time, municipalities grasped the opportunity to use the service housing concept to shift a substantial part of the costs of residential care to the clients and to the state (through sickness insurance). The municipalities also reorganized residential homes as service housing units (Suoniemi, Syrjä, and Taimio 2005).

It has been calculated that during the 1990s municipalities relocated nearly 4000 municipal home-help workers from home-based services to service housing units (MHSA 2004, 25; Vaarama et al. 2001). This implied a major change in the use of personnel resources. This restructuring, together with the fact that the clients who are presently covered by municipal home care need more visits than was previously the case, has meant that the municipalities now provide services to a much smaller proportion of the elderly. By 2003, the percentage of over-75-year-olds receiving regular home help had gone down to 18.7%, from the 31.5% who received help in 1988. The decline for the period 1988–2002 was 40.6 % (MHSA 2006, 176), providing evidence of the rapid narrowing down of public responsibility for elderly home care. In 2004, the Finnish government adopted a rather modest goal according to which elderly home care should cover at least 25% of the elderly over 75 years old (MHSA 2006, 178).

In contrast to the problems of enhancing elderly home care produced by the municipality, the goal of creating a private market was successfully implemented. The number of private providers of home care increased by 70% in the period 1997–2001 and in 2001, the number of private providers rose to 376, of which 70% were firms and 30% voluntary organizations (Finnish Government 2003). This creation of a welfare mix in home care involves care workers both as employees in different kinds of care organizations and as small-scale entrepreneurs (Kovalainen 2004). In 2002, already more than 20% of the care personnel in Finland worked in the private sector, in contrast to less than 13% in the late 1980s (MHSA 2003). This suggests that profound changes have also occurred in the structure of the care work labor market and in employment relations.

The narrowing down of the public responsibility for elderly care was carried out by limiting access to services. A popular way to carry out this task was by classifying clients using indexes based primarily on geriatric knowledge of ageing. Whereas previously elderly people with what were identified as 'medium heavy needs' would mainly have been cared for in residential homes or inpatient primary health care, in the new classification they were to be provided home care with an emphasis on basic care, that is, help with personal bodily care, nutrition or mobility. Those identified as requiring specialized and continuous nursing care were classified as clients with 'heavy needs'. For this group, the policies continued to secure publicly produced care, either in the form of so-called intensified home care or, as a last resort, as residential care. The policies expressed a keen interest in hindering the elderly from turning into clients with 'heavy' needs. Considering this, it is perhaps surprising that after the neo-liberal reforms, the elderly who were considered to have 'light needs' and who would earlier have been eligible for home help, were no longer in any way a public concern (Vaarama et al. 2001).

In contrast to the universalistic era, the policy documents of the early 2000s thus emphasize the last-resort nature of the public services. The role of publicly provided care is often referred to as the provision of temporary solutions, filling in when family care is not adequate or if the care receiver is unable to buy the substitute services from the market (MHSA 2001, 14). The policy rhetoric continued to reduce the traditional homemaking culture by stating that the person, not the home, was to be the focus. The new element is that household chores are not only excluded from the definition of care but reframed as essentially a private concern.

Even though the scope of public elderly care has diminished, and in important ways the public sector has withdrawn from responsibility for older people, the municipalities still have considerable power to regulate the services that they produce. According to the legislation that is currently being implemented, the personnel employed by the private service providers are expected to fulfill qualification criteria corresponding to those required by municipal employees. Additionally, the service providers themselves need to acquire formal approval for their practice from the local authorities. Acquiring such approval presumes that the service provider has not been subject to disciplinary actions for malpractice, or had serious financial difficulties (MHSA 2005, 29–31). The legislation on the supervision of service provision places municipal and other service providers in unequal positions, as the municipality has the authority to issue other service providers permits to operate. Thus it not only controls the market but regulates the activities of the other service providers. By way of contrast, the municipalities themselves are only subjected to retroactive supervision through complaints that citizens can make to the county government.

This is an important issue from the point of view of monitoring the adequacy of the personnel resources and divisions of labor.

The national restructuring of the public sector in the 1990s also concerned the vocational education and qualifications for persons providing elderly care. Most importantly, new occupations were created in the 1990s, reflecting the belief in flexible, trans-sectoral solutions also inspired by lifelong learning agendas of education policy. At the core of the reform was the creation of the *vocational qualification in social and health care*, for which the occupational title is officially translated into English with the term *practical nurse*. Practical nurses are frontline care workers, who as members of a multi-professional team were supposed to provide both socially defined care and general nursing in elderly home care.[5]

The new occupation disrupted the previous division of labor in elderly home care, at least at the level of credentials. Two previously separate educational orientations preparing for care work—one for the social-sector homemakers and the other for the health-sector practical nurses (or auxiliary nurses)—were merged. The new care worker was included in the legislation on the registration of health care professionals as one of the groups authorized to provide nursing care at a level defined by their formal skill and competence.[6] The rhetoric of education policy was to broaden the scope of practice and to reach a better match between education and the labor market (Vuorensyrjä et al. 2006). The policy was aimed at implanting the idea of flexible professionals into the care sector (Wrede 2008). However, in the workplace the occupational roles of the newcomers have remained turbulent.

Though the practical nurse was established as a new care-worker category more than a decade ago, it is still difficult to recruit young people to elderly care. The high levels of drop-outs reflect the mismatch between educational policies and working life practices. The problems of front-line care work have been raised as a national policy concern (MHSA 2001, 2006). The relatively easy access and the shortness of the education, its practical emphasis, and the varying opportunities to obtain partial credentials, tempt policy makers to use the education program as a social policy instrument. Long-term unemployed and other groups, particularly the young and ethnic minorities who for some reason are threatened by marginalization, are directed to the occupation by officials. Research indicates that the young in particular tend to view the occupation of the practical nurse as a temporary, low-paid job that competes poorly with a permanent one with a better salary (Pitkänen 2005).

THE RISE OF THE MEDICO-MANAGERIAL CULTURE

In this section, we draw attention to the implementation of the neo-liberal reforms from two meso-level perspectives. Firstly, we examine the 'rationalization' of municipal home care through policymaking, of which the City of Helsinki is used as an example. Secondly, we study how the trade unions representing health care professionals defend the agency of the care worker.

Implementation of Trans-sectoral Home Care

The national-level institutional restructuring of the welfare state in Finland has resulted in a profound change in the content and scope of elderly home care, speeded up by the lack of resources. We argue that this institutional restructuring at the municipal level is equally profound. In the late 1990s and early 2000s, most municipalities reorganized public home care, and most of the larger cities implemented some 'trans-sectoral' model of elderly home care. This meant that what was earlier known as 'home nursing' emerged as the key element in the new institutional matrix for home care. The emphasis on health care reflects the aim of replacing rather than postponing expensive residential care with the means of elderly home care.

Our previous examination of the home care reform implemented by the City of Helsinki showed concretely how difficult it is to both save money and to carry out a merger of social and health care into one integrated form of service (Wrede and Henriksson 2004). The experiences gained from this restructuring intended to achieve cost-effectiveness show that home care in some cases is more expensive than residential care (see also Ala-Nikkola 2003). Such observations did not, however, disrupt the overall direction of change towards the increasing medicalization of home-based services. In the model that is currently being implemented, the City of Helsinki has gathered different forms of home care for the elderly into one service under the city health authority. The service is however, still divided into three separate streams: home help, home nursing and the intensive home care unit. This three-fold structure also appears as a hierarchy of expertise, and the home care units are expected to function as a part of the so-called care chain in health services.

These changes resulted in significant organizational and cultural constraints for the employees. The new medicalized and managerialist ethos undermined the expertise of frontline carers, even though it is they who directly encounter clients. One of the key reasons for this development was the implementation of a hospital-like hierarchical division of labor in municipal home care. This meant that the frontline care worker was assigned the task of providing only 'basic care', which generally referred to the care of the client's body. The medico-managerial logic is seen in the logistical or task oriented approach to care that results in the omission of socially defined care and the discounting of related skills and competence. Consequently, the social needs of the client were neglected. Practical care work was to be based on general and specialized nursing (Wrede and Henriksson 2004).

Unionist Attempts to Reclaim Professional Mandates in Elderly Care

In the face of managerialist pressures to reorganize welfare services and lower and disrupt occupational boundaries, the trade unions representing care workers appear to share the goal of trying to 'bring the state back' into welfare service policy. The return of the state would mean that the autonomy of the municipality as an employer and a local service producer would be curtailed as a result of the increasing state regulation. In their statements, the unions representing health care occupations have argued that the impending shortage of labor cannot be resolved with what is referred to as local task displacements in national policy agendas. Instead the unions demand national regulation to guarantee the quality of the services and to ensure an 'adequate' division of labor among care professionals, i.e., one that respects traditional occupational boundaries and credentials. Furthermore, the unions attack the municipalities for their 'unethical' employment policies.

The introduction of the 'trans-sectoral' practical nurse has challenged organizational and professional boundaries in many senses. In its response to the new policies, Tehy, the union mainly representing nurses, repeatedly argued for the need to 'respect occupational boundaries'. Apparently, however, an even greater threat than the trans-sectoral occupation for Tehy was the practice of allowing personnel lacking health care qualifications to perform nursing tasks on the basis of workplace level permits. "[The old style] home helpers out of nursing" (Tehy 2003) was a slogan used by the union in a local campaign intended to defend the mandate of nurses.

The trans-sectoral model for organizing elderly home care has, however, also been perceived as a threat by nurses. The loudest reaction against integrated home care came from public health nurses. The union feared that public health nurses would be forced to accept supervision from managers external to their profession, that is, from either nurses or social care professionals. The union further claimed that public health nurse vacancies were abolished and replaced with nurse vacancies, reflecting the marginal role of preventive care in Finnish health policy since the 1990s. Instead of challenging that policy, the union stated that the elderly needed support in the form of health education if they were to be 'active senior citizens'. In addition to what can be characterized as their traditional strategy of referring to their role as experts in health promotion, the union sought to safeguard the jobs and the competence of the public health nurses. The change in their mandates was legalized after "prolonged negotiations" (Terveydenhoitaja 2002). In 2002, the publication jubilantly announced that a new double credential now qualified them both as nurses and as public health nurses, which also followed the EU standards.

Our analysis of the views and claims of the public health nurses' union shows that policy making concerning the public sector workforce often has an indirect impact on the organization of elderly home care. When considering, for instance, recent personnel policy, it is evident that the main attention in the national elderly care policy has focused on nurses and medical doctors. Frontline care workers, such as practical nurses, have hardly been mentioned, except in terms of recruitment problems. The union that represents the majority of practical nurses (SuPer) has frequently tried to draw attention to the mismatch between social policy, labor market policy and education policy, and to the conflicting pressures these policies create when combined with the realities of working life. The major threats to their occupational mandate have derived both from below and from above the occupational hierarchy. Even though the union publication of SuPer constantly raised the problem of inadequate staffing as an important policy concern, its primary interest appeared to be to uphold strict boundaries towards the uneducated care workers. In the early 2000s, SuPer repeatedly claimed that, due to staffing pressures, practical nurses had a hard time in establishing their positions in the labor market and in getting recognition in the workplace. From SuPer's point of view, when "tasks [were] taken from the hands [of practical nurses]" (2002), the problem was that the new trans-sectoral occupation was unknown and the skill and competence undervalued. The pressures from above were related to nurses. Particularly in the late 1990s, public-sector vacancies at this level were replaced with nurse vacancies.

SuPer has tried to improve the position and esteem of the practical nurses. There have been, however, severe obstacles to those pursuits. Firstly, the new vocational qualification was truly non-uniform and, in many cases, uneven. The standardization of education has not been a priority for policymakers. Secondly, SuPer itself has faced internal pressures that have forced its leaders to mediate between, for instance, the former and the new types of practical nurses. SuPer, which was established around one occupation, has faced new challenges to create a united front with the traditional members based in health care and hospital work and the newcomers working in diverse care settings (Henriksson 2008). To succeed, the policy claims of the union need to reflect this diversity; at the same time, it is likely that the internal power relations within the union play a major role in its strategies. This balancing act is probably reflected in the fact that the union has constantly focused more on opposing the devaluation of practical nurses in hospitals than on defending them as providers of socially defined care.

IMPOVERISHMENT OF CARE WORK CULTURE IN ELDERLY HOME CARE

The institutional restructuring of service provision and the narrowing of the scope of public responsibility have contributed towards a welfare mix in home care for the elderly. The strategic role municipal home care now plays differs from the comprehensive responsibility it previously held. The curtailed municipal home care caters to those elderly who have the most severe care needs. The elderly whose care needs are less severe or of the 'wrong kind' are of no concern to the public sector. Public services now aim at providing a last resort scheme, basic service for the sickest elderly, rather than universal service available to all citizens on the basis of care needs. Regulatory changes reflect a new definition of the division of labor among the state, the market and the family. What has resulted is an increasingly medicalized public service along with a non-uniform mix of diverse service settings and care work cultures.

In the resulting institutional matrix, the frontline care workers in public elderly care have lost their license to provide socially defined care. The power to organize everyday care has been transferred to the managerial elite and to the politicians in the municipalities. The care workers who provide socially defined care appear to be the biggest losers when their room to define and to control their work is considered.

The discussion about the views and strategies of the unions of care workers illustrates the disconnectedness of their responses to the restructuring of elderly care. The wave of neo-liberal policies that is here characterized as the introduction of a medico-managerialist care culture in public elderly home care appears to have contributed to the polarization of care workers and the fragmentation of their organizations. As a result of deregulation, the diverse groups who carry out socially defined care in non-public organizational settings have disintegrated. A new distribution of employment opportunities can be discerned between those who work in the regulated outsourced services and those who work in services that clients purchase directly from the market.

The emerging social order in Finnish public home care for the elderly is one that has been reorganized along the cultural order of 'upstairs and downstairs' in which only the upstairs is entitled to professionalism (Wrede and Henriksson 2004). Thus, the implementation of the neo-liberal elderly care reforms created inequalities in the division of labor through evoking traditional professionalism with its divisive, conservative and individualistic tones (Henriksson, Wrede and Burau 2006). Implementation of the medico-managerial care culture in the public elderly home care has strengthened the position of the key experts, the medical doctors and nurses, whereas the competence in socially defined care that practical nurses partly represent is not recognized. To be sure, practical nurses are registered health care professionals authorized to provide general nursing care, but their skill and competence in *social care* are challenged, excluded and devalued.

By reconfiguring the skill and competence in public home care for the elderly, policy makers have set up a hierarchical and task-oriented care work culture. The restructuring of home care has resulted in an *institutional* devaluation of socially defined care. Despite the educational ideals and the policy rhetoric, career opportunities have appeared only for the more educated professionals, for instance, as managers or specialized experts. In contrast, the autonomy available to frontline workers in their practical everyday work is curtailed. The organization further blurs their work role through an unclear system of task transferrals. The lack of recognition of the occupational or organizational license to perform nursing tasks appears to be a constant cause for conflicts in the workplace.

A further structural hindrance to stable work roles for practical nurses has been the high prevalence of temporary contracts. Benefiting from the high unemployment rates of the recession years in the 1990s, municipalities created a buffer of the temporary workforce in the public sector. The large group of temporary care workers had poor employment rights and few opportunities to develop their skill and competence. These terms and conditions restricted the autonomy and agency of the frontline workers. In turn, these processes also seemed to generate other pressures, including recruitment problems and boundary struggles for unions. Probably the most severe threat caused by this lack of recognition from the perspective of the frontline care workers, is the related crisis of professional commitment and identity that increasingly seems to frighten away potential recruits, especially young people.

As discussed above, *geriatrics* rather than gerontology has emerged as the new core expertise in municipal home care, both at the municipal level and in the national planning of cost-effective elderly care policy. Policymakers are prone to look for answers to the problems identified in elderly care in health care expertise in general and geriatrics in particular. This is demonstrated by one of the policy documents that focused on the need to intensify the medical contribution in elderly care (MHSA 2006). Not surprisingly, the rapporteur recommends the promotion of education and knowledge formation in the subspecialties of geriatrics, such as geriatric psychiatry and pharmaceutical medicine.

In this chapter, we have shown how the care-friendly and the care worker-friendly universalistic welfare state became questioned and dismantled through the neo-liberal policies implemented since the 1990s. In the reformed institutional matrix, care and economic efficiency are constantly juxtaposed, giving superiority to the latter. When analyzing the developments resulting from this austere neo-liberal ethos, we underline the ideological chasm between the care-friendly welfare state with its democratic professionalism and the cost-controlling state with its elitist professionalism. In the face of the emerging inequalities in relation to the eligibility for public services and in occupational and employment opportunities for care workers evident in the Finnish society as well as globally, we suggest that researchers, policy makers and citizens once again become concerned about social justice and the equal distribution of resources. Such concerns entail posing questions similar to those once so potently posed by feminist scholars of the 1970s and the 1980s, at the same time taking into consideration the increasing complexity of our societies.

NOTES

1. Originally published in 2008 in *Care Work in Crisis. Reclaiming the Nordic Ethos of Care*, edited by Sirpa Wrede, Lea Henriksson, H. Høst, S. Johansson and B. Dybbroe. Lund, Sweden: Studentlitteratur. Reprinted with permission from Studentlitteratur.
2. This chapter develops empirical analysis earlier reported in Henriksson and Wrede 2004, Wrede and Henriksson 2004, 2005 and Henriksson, Wrede and Burau 2006. These publications include a more detailed empirical analysis of the documents used.
3. The set of documents was mainly collected for the Academy of Finland project *Service Professions in Transition* (2001–2004). The documents had three foci, national policy, local policy in the city of Helsinki and a discussion of home care in the trade union publications of occupations in the health care sector. At the national level, we privileged policy documents originating from state policy actors. At the local level, our materials originated from one central project of elderly care reform. It was governed by the social authority in the local context, but the central experts in the project group were primarily health care professionals. Our choice of trade union publications excluded trade unions that exclusively represent social care occupations. The systematic review of the union publications covered the years 2000–2004 and the review of the Helsinki policy documents the period 2002–2004. Later, we collected diverse materials on elderly home care in two Academy of Finland projects: *The Politics of Recruitment* (Henriksson) and *The New Dynamics of Professionalism within Caring Occupations* (Wrede).
4. In the early 2000's, there were more than 400 municipalities in Finland. These varied greatly in size, economic capacity, demographic structure and the service needs of the population. Currently, a major structural reform is being carried out that substantially cut the number of municipalities. In 2011, their number is 336.
5. A trans-sectoral occupation was also created for the administration of elderly care. In English, the program is called a 'Degree Program in Human Ageing and Elderly Service' (occupational title in Swedish *geronom*). This degree corresponds to the nursing and social work programs which all are offered at the polytechnics. '*Geronoms*' remain rare in elderly care administration. Apparently, many of them work in tasks below their educational level, for instance, as practical nurses (Kuntalehti 2007). They are not, however, registered as health care professionals and therefore lack the formal qualification required for nursing tasks (Supreme Administrative Court 2006).
6. Health care professionals are described in the Act (559/1994) and Decree (564/1994) on Health Care Professionals. Health care professionals include a) licensed professionals, b) professionals having a permit, c) professionals with a protected occupational title. Registration as a health care professional is the basic requirement for many nursing tasks and for the provision of medical care.

REFERENCES

Ala-Nikkola, Merja. 2003. *Sairaalassa, kotona vai vanhainkodissa?* Acta Universitatis Tamperensis 972. Tampere: University of Tampere.
Borgman, Merja. 1998. *Miten sosiaalialan työntekijöiden ammatilliset tulkinnat rakentuvat?* Helsinki: Stakes, Tutkimuksia 95.

Finnish Government. 2003. *Hallituksen esitys Eduskunnalle laeiksi sosiaali- ja terveydenhuollon suunnittelusta ja valtionosuudesta annetun lain 4 §:n, sosiaalihuoltolain sekä sosiaali- ja terveydenhuollon asiakasmaksuista annetun lain 12 §:n muuttamisesta. HE 74/2003.*

Freeman, Richard. 1999. Institutions, states and cultures: Health policy and politics in Europe. In *Comparative social policy. Concepts, theories and methods,* edited by Jochen Clasen, 80–94. Oxford: Blackwell Publishers.

Henriksson, Lea. 2008. Reconfiguring Finnish welfare service workforce: inequalities and identity. *Equal Opportunities International,* 27 (1): 49–63.

Henriksson, Lea and Sirpa Wrede. Editors. 2004. *Hyvinvointityön ammatit.* Tampere: Vastapaino.

Henriksson, Lea, Sirpa Wrede, and Viola Burau. 2006. Understanding professional projects in welfare service work: revival of old professionalism? *Gender, Work and Organization,* 13(2): 174–192.

Julkunen, Raija. 1994. Hyvinvointivaltiollisten professioprojektin katkos. *Tiede & Edistys,* 19(3): 200–213.

——— 2001. *Suunnanmuutos.* Tampere: Vastapaino.

Koskinen, Simo, Seija Ahonen, Marja Jylhä, Anna-Liisa Korhonen and Marita Paunonen. 1988. *Vanhustyö.* Helsinki: Vanhustyön keskusliitto.

Kovalainen, Anne. 2004. Hyvinvointipalvelujen markkinoituminen ja sukupuolisopimuksen muutos. In *Hyvinvointityön ammatit,* edited by Lea Henriksson and Sirpa Wrede, 187–209. Tampere: Vastapaino.

Kröger, Teppo, Anneli Anttonen and Jorma Sipilä. 2003. Social care in Finland: Stronger and weaker forms of universalism. In *The Young, the Old and the State. Social Care Systems in Five Industrial Nations,* edited by Anneli Anttonen, John Baldock, and Jorma Sipilä, 25–54. Cheltenham: Edward Elgar.

Kuntalehti. 2007. Geronomi on vanhustyön ammattilainen. February 7: 3, 47.

MHSA. 2001. *Sosiaali- ja terveydenhuollon työvoimatarpeen ennakointitoimikunnan mietintö.* Komiteanmietintö 2001:7. Helsinki: Ministry of Health and Social Affairs.

MHSA. 2003. Ailasmaa, Reijo. Sosiaali- ja terveydenhuollon työvoiman ja koulutuksen ennakoinnin työryhmä. *Kuntien sosiaali- ja terveydenhuollon henkilöstö 1990–2001.* (Retrieved 2003–10–15.) www.stm.fi/Resource.phx/hankk/hankt/ennakointi/tyovoima.htx.i1535.ppt

MHSA. 2004. *Valtakunnallinen omaishoidon uudistaminen.* Selvityshenkilö Elli Aaltosen ehdotukset. Working group reports 2004:3. Helsinki: Ministry of Health and Social Affairs.

MHSA. 2005. *Palveluseteli. Käyttöopas kotipalveluun.* Sosiaali- ja terveysministeriön oppaita 2005:1. Helsinki: Ministry of Health and Social Affairs.

MHSA. 2006. *Geriatrisen hoidon ja vanhustyön kehittäminen.* Sosiaali- ja terveysministeriön selvityksiä 30/2006. Selvityshenkilö Sirkka-Liisa Kivelä. Helsinki: Ministry of Health and Social Affairs.

Paasivaara, Leena. 2002. *Suomalaisen vanhusten hoitotyön muotoutuminen monitasotarkastelussa 1930-luvulta 2000-luvulle.* Oulu: Oulun yliopisto.

Pitkänen, Marita. 2005. Raskasta mutta antoisaa. Työvoimapoliittiseen vanhustyön koulutukseen osallistuneiden käsityksiä vanhustyöstä. Unpublished master's thesis. Tampere: University of Tampere, Department of Social Policy and Social Work.

Rauhala, Pirkko-Liisa. 1996. Sosiaalipalvelut käytäntönä. In *Sosiaalipalvelujen Suomi,* edited by Jorma Sipilä, Outi Ketola, Teppo Kröger and Pirkko-Liisa Rauhala, 121–155. Juva: WSOY.

Simonen, Leila. 1990. *Contradictions of the welfare state, women and caring. Municipal home making in Finland.* Tampere: Acta Universitatis Tamperensis ser A vol 2. 95.

SuPer. 2002. Välittäminen on elämän perusvoima. Juhani Palomäki asiaa johtamisesta. *49(2): 3.*

Supreme Administrative Court. 2006. Kunnallisasia—Työsopimussuhteinen toimi—Toimen täyttäminen—Kelpoisuus—Lähihoitaja—Hallintolainkäyttöasia. *KHO: 2006:28.* Helsinki: Korkein hallinto-oikeus.

Suoniemi, Ilpo, Vesa Syrjä and Heikki Taimio. 2005. *Vanhusten asumispalvelujen kilpailuttaminen.* Tutkimuksia No. 97. Helsinki: Palkansaajien tutkimuslaitos.

Tedre, Silva. 1999. *Hoivan sanattomat sopimukset. Tutkimus vanhusten kotipalvelun työntekijöiden työstä.* Joensuu: Joensuun yliopiston yhteiskuntatieteellisiä julkaisuja 40.

———— 2004. Likainen työ ja virallinen hoiva. In *Hyvinvointityön ammatit,* edited by Lea Henriksson and Sirpa Wrede, 63–83. Tampere: Vastapaino.

Tehy. 2003. Kotiavustajat pois sairaanhoidosta. 22:11, 29.

Terveydenhoitaja. 2002 Terveydenhoitajat laillistetaan nyt myös sairaanhoitajina. 35:8, 6.

Vaarama, Marja, Jaakko Luomahaara, Arja Peiponen and Päivi Voutilainen. 2001. *Koko kunta ikääntyneiden asialle.* Raportteja 259. Helsinki: Stakes.

Vaarama, Marja and Anja Noro. 2005. Vanhusten palvelut. *Duodecim Terveyskirjasto.* Retrieved 2011–05–23. http://www.terveyskirjasto.fi/terveyskirjasto/tk.koti?p_artikkeli=suo00058.

Vuorensyrjä, Matti, Merja Borgman, Tarja Kemppainen, Mikko Mäntysaari and Anneli Pohjala. 2006. *Sosiaalialan osaajat 2015. Sosiaalialan osaamis-, työvoima- ja koulutustarpeiden ennakointihanke (SOTENNA): loppuraportti.* Jyväskylä: Opetusministeriö, Euroopan Sosiaalirahasto, Sosiaali- ja terveysministeriö, Suomen Kuntaliitto.

Waerness, Kari. 1984. Caring as women's work in the welfare state. In *Patriarchy in a welfare society,* edited by Harriet Holter, 67–87. Oslo: Universitetsforlaget.

———— 1992. Bettering the public care services—the only realistic alternative for strengthening the welfare of ordinary people in need of care. In *Sosiaalipalvelujen kehitystrendejä eri maissa,* edited by Jorma Sipilä, 98–124. Tampere: University of Tampere.

Wrede, Sirpa. 2008. Educating generalists: Flexibility and identity in auxiliary nursing in Finland. In *Rethinking professional governance. International directions in health care,* edited by Ellen Kuhlmann and Mike Saks, 127–140. Brisol: Policy Press.

Wrede, Sirpa and Lea Henriksson. 2004. Kahden kerroksen väkeä: Kotihoidon ammatillinen uusjako. In *Hyvinvointityön ammatit,* edited by Lea Henriksson and SirpaWrede, 210–234. Tampere: Vastapaino.

———— 2005. The changing terms of welfare service work: Finnish home care in transition. In *Dilemmas of care in the Nordic welfare state. Continuity and change,* edited by Hanne Marlene Dahl and Tina Rask Eriksen, 62–79. Aldershot: Ashgate.

Contributors

Davina Allen is Professor in the Cardiff School of Nursing and Midwifery Studies at Cardiff University, Wales, UK.

Kristin Björnsdóttir is Professor in the Faculty of Nursing, School of Health Sciences at the University of Iceland, Iceland.

Christine Ceci is Assistant Professor in the Faculty of Nursing at the University of Alberta, Canada.

Hanne Marlene Dahl is Professor in the Department of Society and Globalisation at Roskilde University, Denmark.

Isabel Dyck is Professor in the School of Geography at Queen Mary, University of London, UK.

Kim England is Professor in the Department of Geography at University of Washington–Seattle, USA.

Lea Henriksson is Adjunct Professor and Senior Research Fellow in the University of Tampere Centre for Advanced Study (UTACAS) at University of Tampere, Finland.

Joanna Latimer is Professor in the Cardiff University School of Social Sciences at Cardiff University, Wales, UK.

Carl May is Professor of Healthcare Innovation and Associate Dean, Research in the Faculty of Health Sciences at University of Southampton, UK.

Anna Olaison is Senior Lecturer, NISAL (National Institute for the Study of Ageing and Later Life) at Campus Norrköping at Linköping University, Sweden.

Mary Ellen Purkis is Dean and Professor in the Faculty of Human and Social Development at University of Victoria, Canada.

Sirpa Wrede is Professor in the Department of Social Research / Sociology at University of Helsinki, Finland.

Index